COOK IT UP

Delicious recipes for healthy cooking

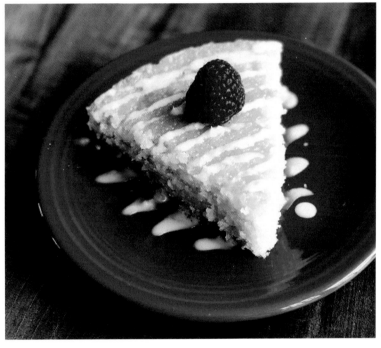

To Samantha
Cook It Up!
Catherine
Walker

CATHERINE WALKER

Every recipe in this book is dairy, egg, peanut & tree nut free

Published by Baker and Taylor's Bookbaby
7905 North Crescent Boulevard
Pennsauken, New Jersey 08110

ISBN: 978-1-54393-139-6

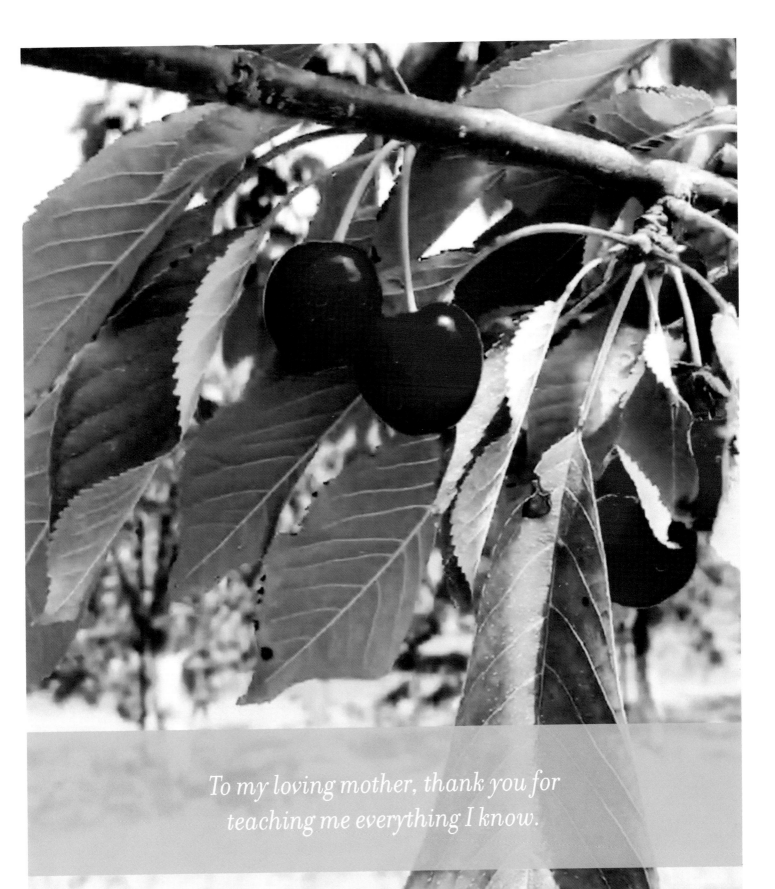

To my loving mother, thank you for teaching me everything I know.

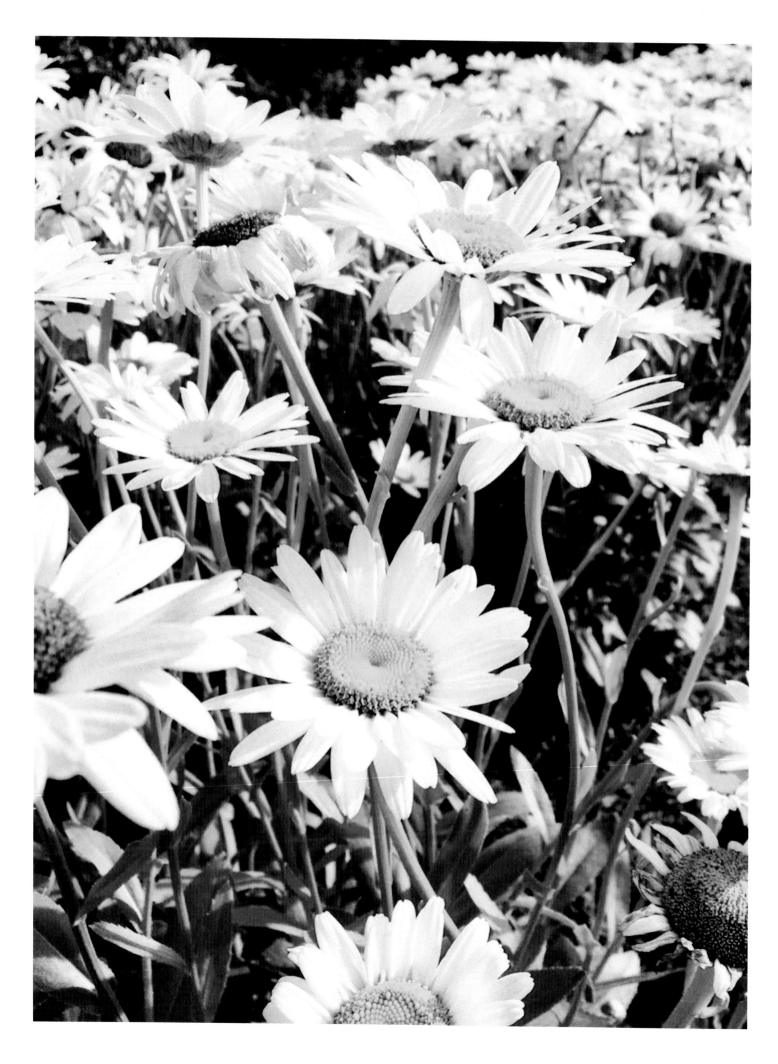

Contents

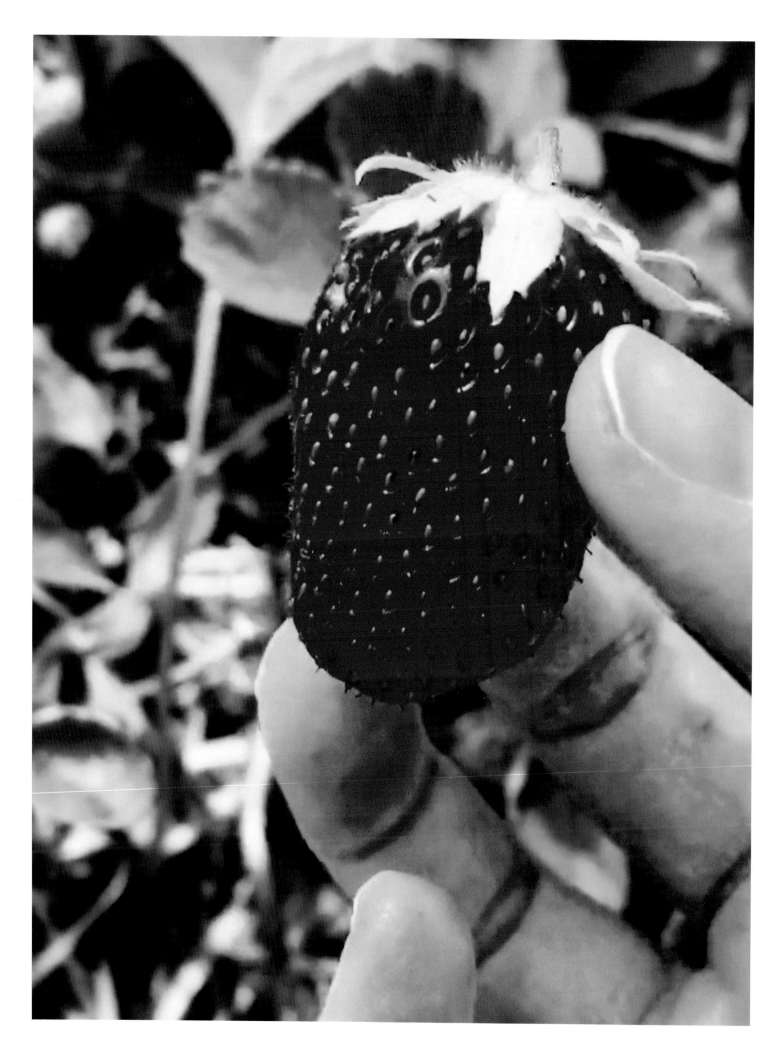

Thank You

Thank you to my entire family for supporting me when I wanted to publish a cookbook. Your love and encouragement helped me present this book to the world.

Thank you to L+P Design and Architecture for designing this cookbook. Your design expertise was invaluable to me and I really enjoyed working with your firm.

Thank you to Old Trail School and all of the teachers who have encouraged me to follow my dream of publishing a cookbook.

Thank you to my advisor Laurie Arnold for guiding me along the way.

A special thank you to my art teachers, Jeff Eason and Patty Wyman who inspire me everyday to be the artist that I am, and for teaching me about art, which always brings a smile to my face.

Thank you to Kathy Sapienza and Alice Goumas for creating Edible Education at Old Trail School which has allowed me to cook at school.

Lastly, thank you to my Hudson friends who have tasted my recipes and provided feedback about them.

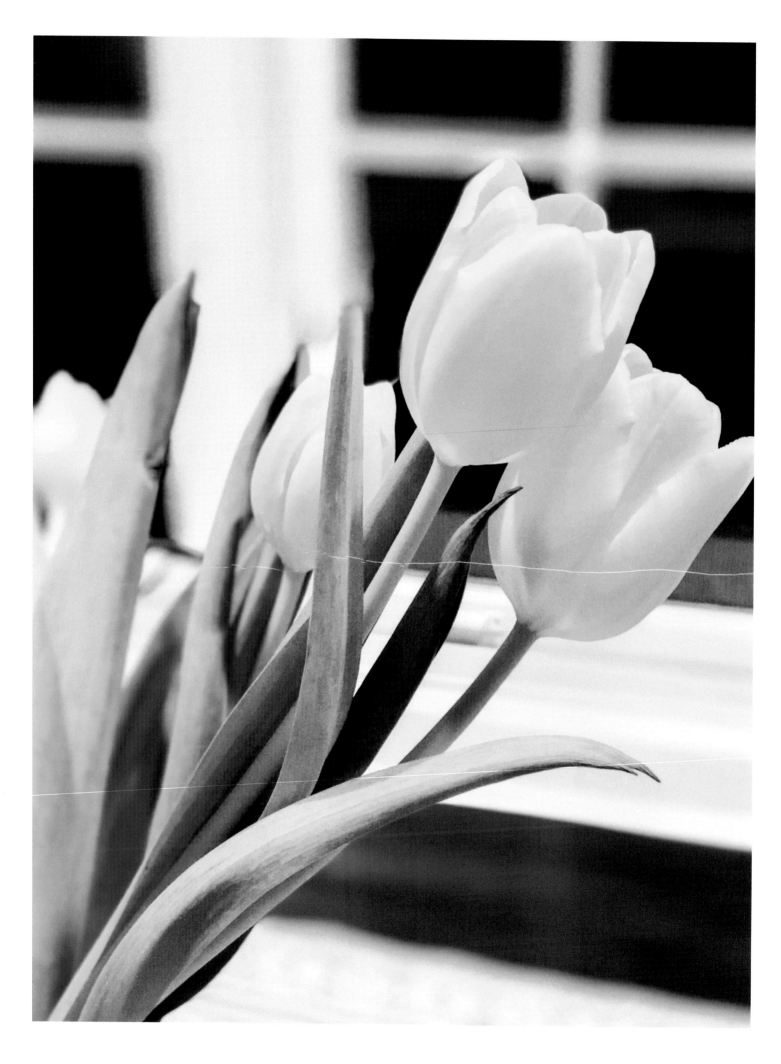

Introduction

This book was written for all of the kids and families with allergies. This book is meant to help them find their way in the kitchen with allergies. I am proud to say that all of my recipes are completely dairy, egg, peanut, and tree nut free. I hope these recipes are as successful and delicious to you as they are to me. When you read these recipes, I believe they will leave your mouth watering because you want to start to Cook It Up. I love cooking these foods, and I encourage you to try to make them yourself and enjoy the wonders of cooking.

Cooking to me is more than just throwing a bunch of ingredients together. It is a part of my heart. All of the recipes that I create are full of thought out flavors, aromas, and ingredients. Cooking is more than a day to day chore — it is a talent passed on from one generation to the next. Cooking is a part of me and so are my recipes. I hope when you cook these recipes, you think about all of the meaning that was put into them and savor the wonderful foods that make cooking delicious and healthy, too.

~ Catherine Walker

Hors D'oeuvres

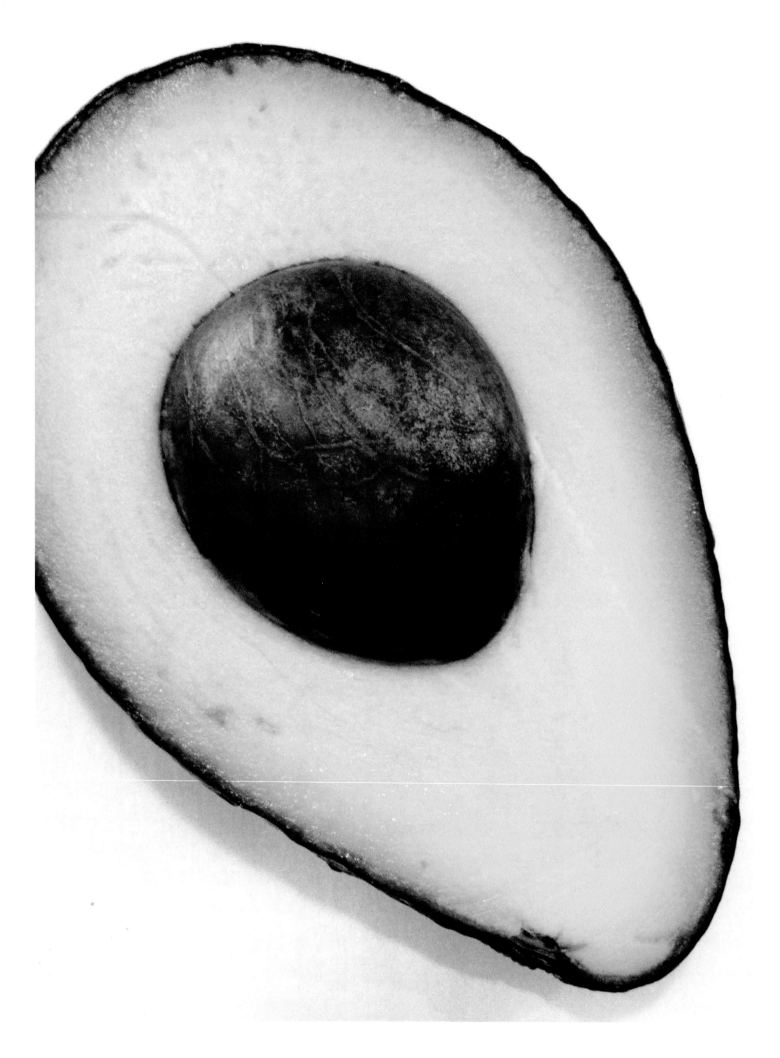

Avocado Spread

1 avocado
1 tablespoon canola oil
2 teaspoons lemon juice (optional)
Pinch of salt

Put everything in a food processor and blend until smooth. Transfer into a bowl. Serve at room temperature with tortilla chips.

Avocado Salsa Verde

4 avocados, finely diced
¼ tomatillo, diced
¼ small white onion, minced
1 teaspoon lime zest
Juice of 1 lime
Juice of ½ lemon
3 tablespoons olive oil
1 tablespoon fresh cilantro, minced
1 garlic clove, minced
2½ teaspoons green hot sauce
1 teaspoon jalapeño, minced
1 jalapeño cut into circles (for garnish)

Transfer the avocados, tomatillos, onion, lime zest, fresh lime juice, fresh lemon juice, olive oil, fresh cilantro, garlic, hot sauce, and minced jalapeño into the bowl of a food processor. Pulse until smooth but still chunky. Garnish with the jalapeño circles and more cilantro. Serve with corn chips on the side.

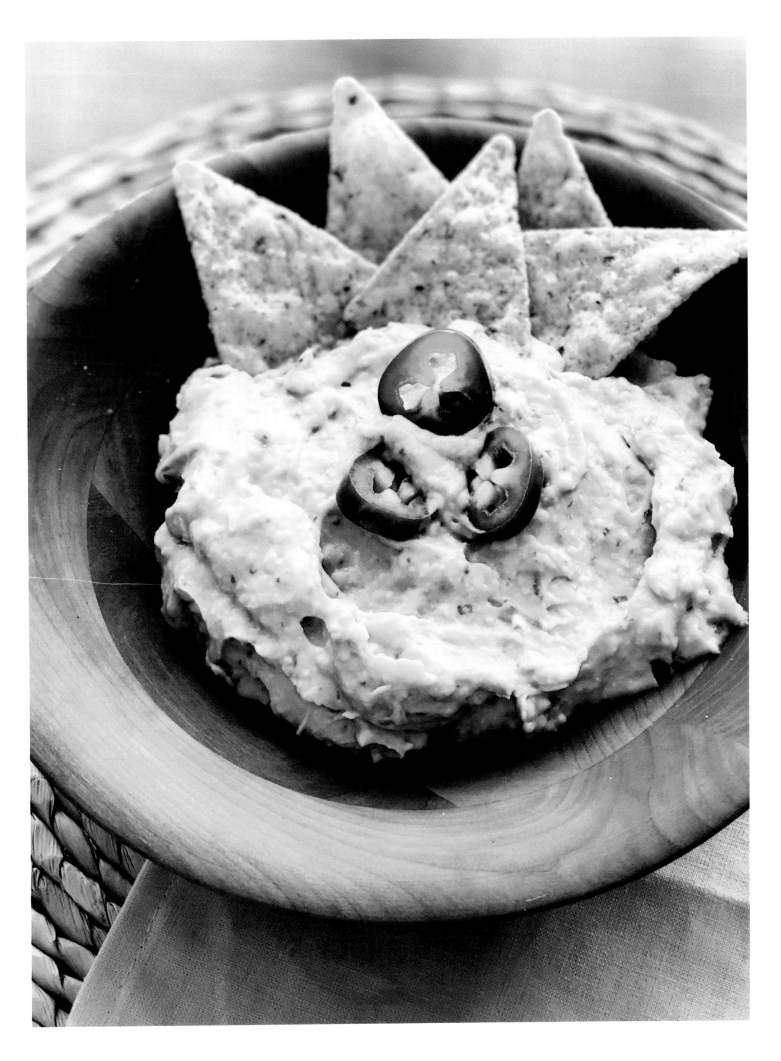

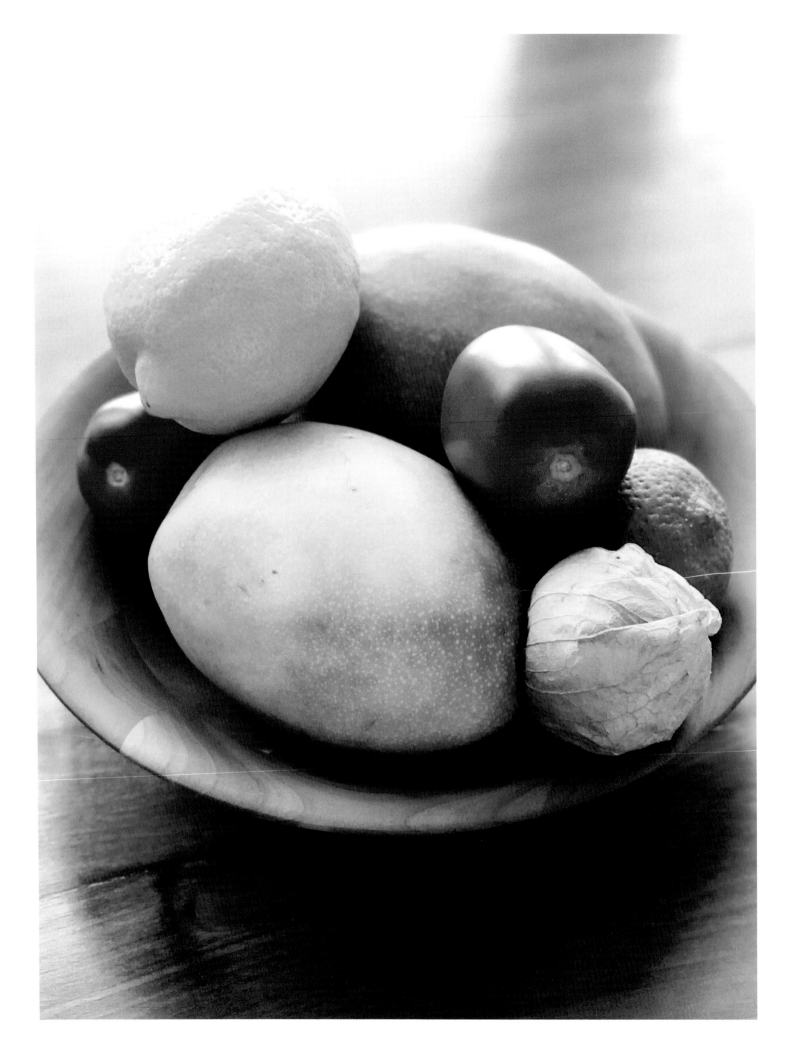

Spicy Mango Salsa

3 fresh mangoes, cubed
1 tomatillo, chopped
½-1 Roma tomato, seeded and diced
1 jalapeño, seeded and chopped
1 garlic clove, minced
Juice of 1 lime
Zest of 1 lime
½ teaspoon chili powder
1 tablespoon fresh lemon juice
2 tablespoons fresh cilantro
Salt
Pepper

Put everything in the bowl of a food processor and pulse until medium chunky. Serve chilled or at room temperature with tortilla chips (store bought or homemade recipe found on page 28).

Bean Dip Base

2 cans Cannellini beans (14 ounce each), rinsed
Salt
Pepper
Olive oil (until it is smooth consistently)

Blend in a food processor until smooth. Chill when not using.

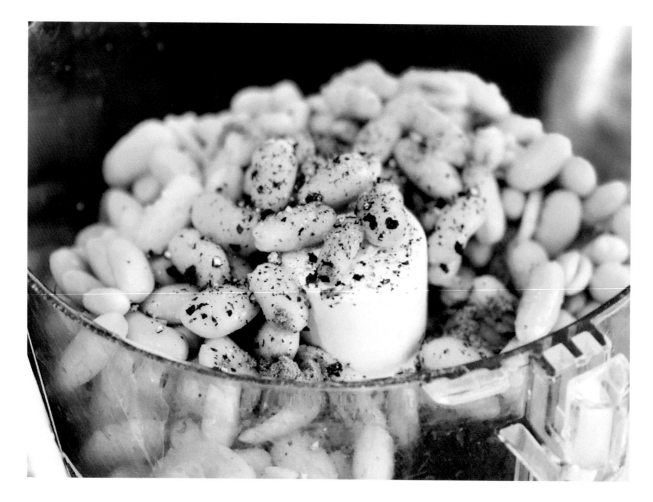

Classic Bean Dip

1 recipe Bean Dip Base (recipe on page 18)

1 tablespoon chives (dried or fresh)

½ teaspoon cumin

½ teaspoon chili powder

1 teaspoon white onions (cooked or dried)

Combine in food processor until smooth. Serve with crackers. Chill.

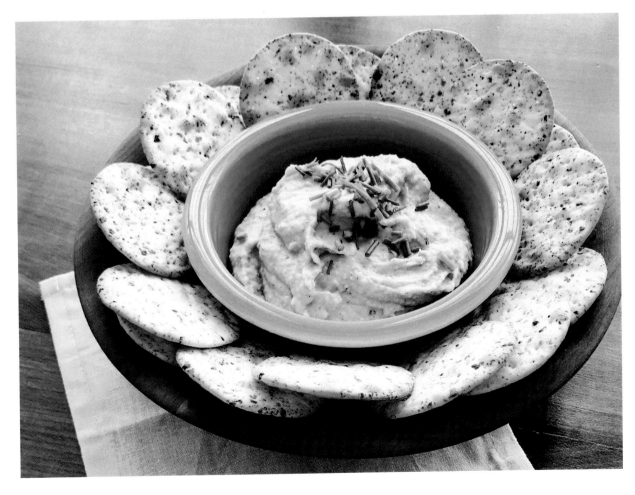

Spiced Red Pepper Hummus

1 recipe Bean Dip Base (recipe on page 18)
1 ancient sweet pepper, seeded and cut into medium size pieces
1 teaspoon chili powder
¼ teaspoon dried minced onion
1 teaspoon smoked paprika

Roast the peppers drizzled with 1 tablespoon olive oil on a sheet pan lined with foil for 20 to 25 minutes at 425 degrees until heavily charred. In the bowl of a food processor, make one recipe of the Bean Dip Base (recipe on page 18), add the chili powder, paprika, onion, and roasted red peppers. Pulse until smooth. Serve with raw veggies or crackers. Chill when not using.

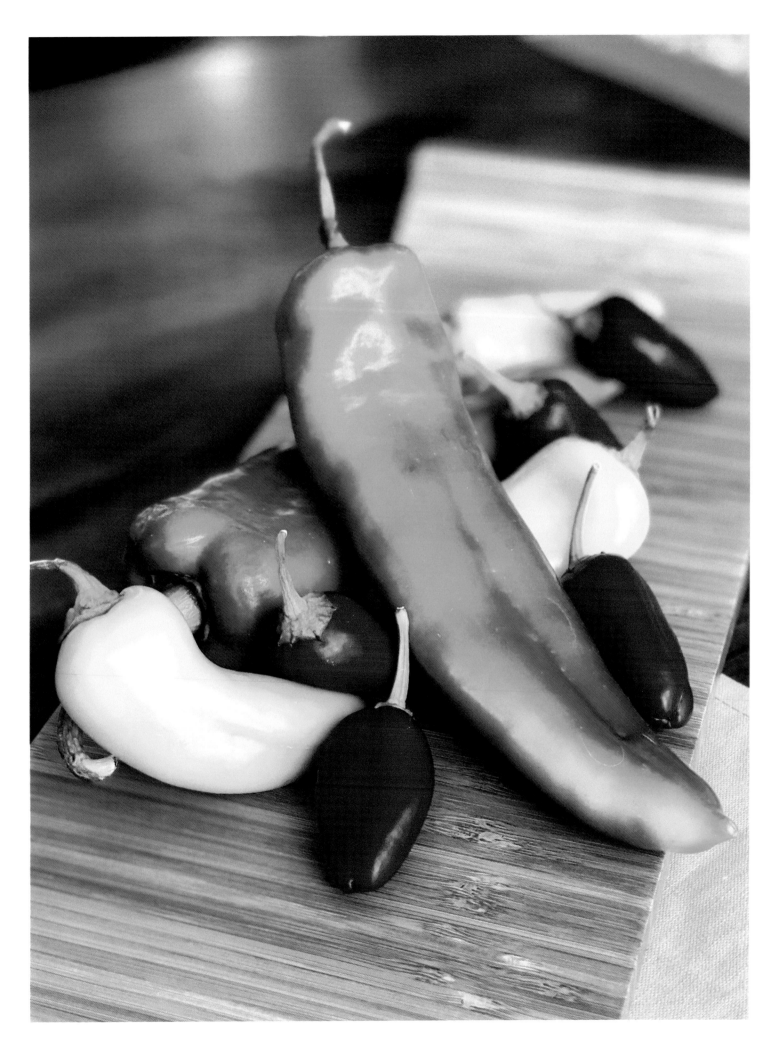

Sun-dried Tomato Basil Dip

1 recipe Bean Dip Base (recipe on page 18)
3 tablespoons sun dried tomatoes (from oil)
4 basil leaves
1 tablespoon chopped, cooked yellow onion.

Blend in a food processor until smooth. Serve cold on a crostini. Chill.

Sweet & Spicy Sweet Potato Dip

1 recipe Bean Dip Base (recipe on page 18)
½ sweet potato, peeled
1 teaspoon honey
⅛ teaspoon cayenne pepper
1 teaspoon cumin
1 tablespoon olive oil
Salt
Pepper

Preheat oven to 400°.

Meanwhile, roughly cut the peeled sweet potato transfer to a sheet pan lined with foil. Drizzle with olive oil and sprinkle with the cayenne, cumin, salt, and pepper. Bake for 10 to 20 minutes until you can poke it with a fork.

Transfer into the food processor and blend with the bean dip base and honey until smooth. Serve with crackers and vegetables. Chill when not using.

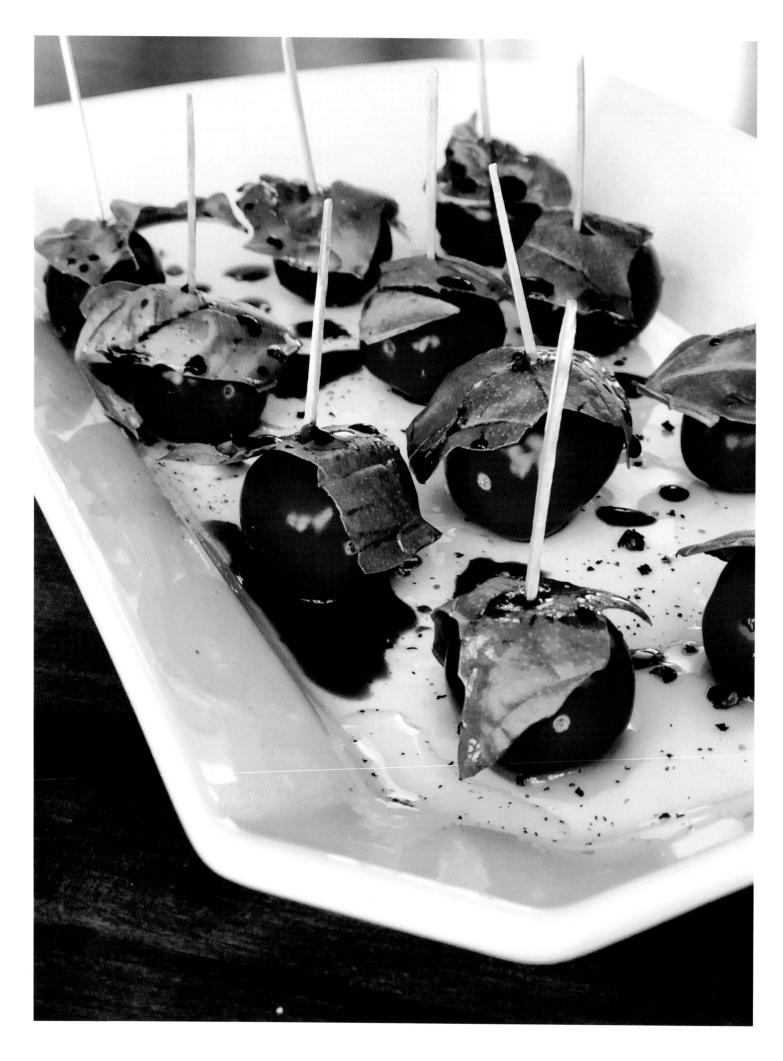

Tomato Basil Toothpicks

2 pints grape tomatoes
15 basil leaves
Balsamic reduction
Olive oil
Freshly ground black pepper
Sea salt

Wash and dry the tomatoes and basil. Tear the basil into medium sized pieces. Poke a grape tomato on it's long side with a toothpick, allowing it to stand up without the toothpick poking through the other end. Layer a piece of basil over the tomato like a blanket. Repeat this process until there are no more tomatoes left. Line up on a platter and drizzle with the balsamic reduction and olive oil. Sprinkle with salt and pepper. Chill.

Breadsticks

2 packages puff pastry
Olive oil (as needed)
Dried thyme
Salt
Freshly ground black pepper
Garlic powder

Preheat oven to 400°.

Roll out puff pastry and cut into 6 x 1 inch strips. Transfer to sheet pan lined with parchment paper. Brush each strip with olive oil and then sprinkle seasonings on top. Bake for 10 to 15 minutes or until golden brown and crisp. Serve warm.

Spinach Mushroom Bites

1 roll Phyllo dough
12 ounces frozen spinach
8 ounces baby Portobello mushrooms
1 tablespoon olive oil
2 teaspoons dairy-free butter
Salt
Pepper
1 garlic clove

Preheat oven to 350°.

Cook the mushrooms with the olive oil, butter, salt, pepper, and garlic. Once the mushrooms are fully cooked, add the spinach and cook until it is wilted.

Transfer into a bowl, set aside. Prepare the phyllo dough as the package says. Cut into long 3 inch strips layer 3 on top of each other, spoon a spoonful of the mushrooms and spinach, fold over to make a triangle. Repeat this step until you are out of the filling. Cook in a preheated oven at 350 degrees for 10 to 15 minutes or until golden brown and crisp. Serve warm dipped in melted butter.

Chili Corn Tortilla Chips

8 corn tortillas, cut into fourths
3 tablespoons olive oil
1 teaspoon salt
½ teaspoon freshly ground black pepper
½ teaspoon fresh lime juice
1 teaspoon chili powder (optional)

Preheat oven to 350°.

Lay the tortillas on a baking sheet in one layer. Mix together the olive oil and lime juice and drizzle on the tortillas. Sprinkle with the salt, pepper, and chili powder. Cook at 350 degrees until golden brown and crisp (about 12 to 15 min). Finish by sprinkling the chips with more salt, pepper, and chili powder. Serve warm or at room temperature.

Easy Thyme Potato Chips

2 Idaho potatoes
Olive oil
Salt
Freshly ground black pepper
Dried thyme

Preheat oven to 400°.

Peel potatoes, and cut into ¼ inch thick slices. Spread out the potatoes on two trays lined with aluminum foil. Drizzle the olive oil over the potatoes. Sprinkle the salt, pepper, and thyme over the potatoes and toss lightly. Cook 20 to 25 minutes until browned and crispy. Serve warm.

Soups & Salads

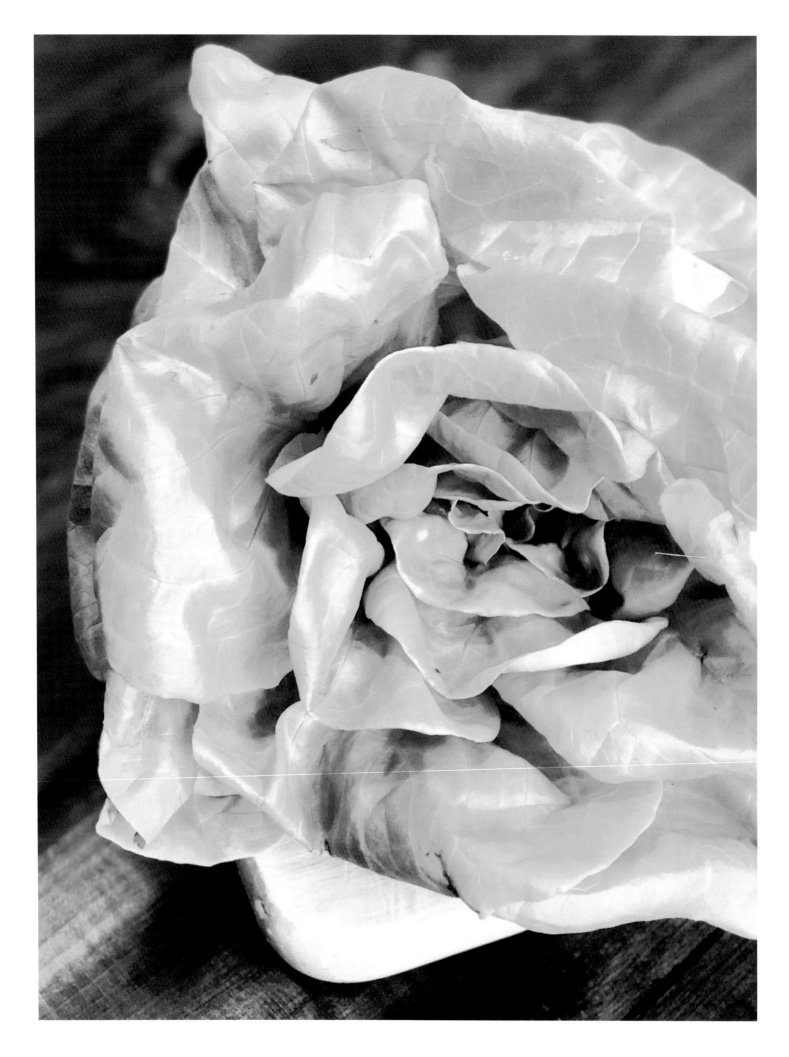

Simple Salad with Balsamic Vinaigrette

1-2 heads of your favorite lettuce, leaves torn
1 Honeycrisp apple, sliced into thin pieces
1 avocado, chopped into cubes
1 cup croutons (homemade or store bought)

FOR THE DRESSING:
½ cup olive oil
3½ tablespoons balsamic vinegar
2 teaspoons honey
1 teaspoon Dijon mustard
1 teaspoon lemon juice
Salt
Freshly ground black pepper

Toss lettuce, apple, avocado and croutons together in a bowl, and set aside. In a separate bowl, whisk the vinaigrette ingredients together. Pour over salad, and toss once more. Serve fresh.

Arugula Salad

2 tablespoons lemon juice
4 tablespoons olive oil
2 cups baby arugula
¼ red onion
2 ears fresh corn

Boil the corn in a big pot on medium-high heat for approximately 5 minutes or until cooked thoroughly. Cut the corn off the cob and set aside. Chop the red onion very finely and mix with the corn. Toss everything together in a big bowl. Serve at room temperature.

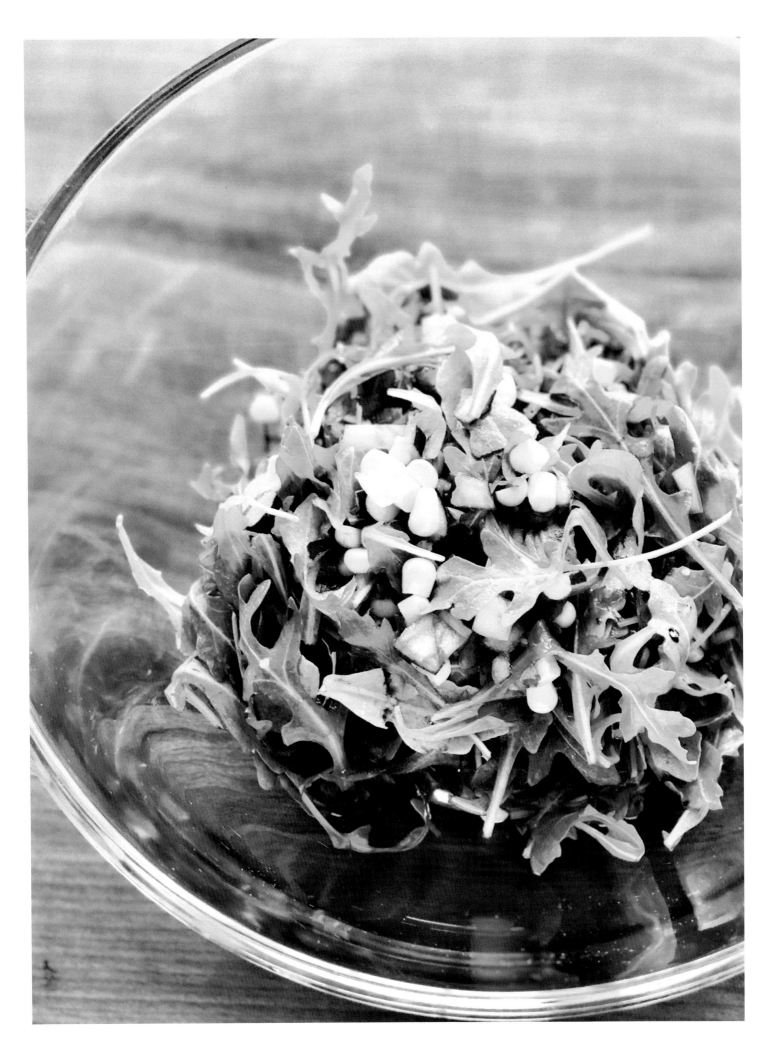

Summer Super Salad

2 heads small leaf lettuce
¼ cup olive oil
1 pint grape tomatoes
½ medium white onion
1 avocado
1 red apple
½ cup cooked bacon, crumbled
3 ears cooked corn
Salt, to taste
Freshly ground black pepper
¼ teaspoon chili powder

FOR THE DRESSING:
½ cup olive oil
3½ tablespoons balsamic vinegar
1 teaspoon Dijon mustard
Salt
Freshly ground black pepper

Whisk the olive oil, balsamic vinegar, mustard, salt and pepper in a small bowl. Set aside for later.

Place the lettuce in a big bowl. Then, in a large sauté pan, cook the whole grape tomatoes with some olive oil, a spoonful of the dressing, salt, and pepper until tender (don't let them pop open). Transfer the tomatoes into the bowl of lettuce. Roughly chop the onions into half circles. In the same sauté pan used to cook tomatoes, cook the onions with more olive oil, salt, pepper, and chili powder. Cook the onions until almost transparent. Transfer the onions into the lettuce making sure to get all of the oil left in the pan. Cube the avocado and add it to the lettuce. Chop the apple into thin strips (you can keep the skin on peel if preferred). Add the apples to the salad. Crumble the bacon and cut the corn off the cob. Then, transfer everything into the salad. Finally dress with dressing and toss. Add Crunchy Thyme Croutons (recipe on page 47). Serve at room temperature or chilled.

Arugula Apple Salad

12 ounces fresh arugula
5 Granny Smith apples, diced
1 cup crumbled, cooked bacon
1 small yellow onion, chopped
1 teaspoon apple cider vinegar
1 teaspoon brown sugar
2 tablespoons canola or olive oil

FOR THE DRESSING:
2 tablespoons apple cider vinegar
¾ cup olive or canola oil
¼ teaspoon cumin
1 tablespoon fresh thyme leaves
Salt
Pepper

For the dressing, in a medium bowl, mix together the apple cider vinegar, oil, cumin, thyme, salt, and pepper. Chill for 5 to 10 minutes. Dress over the salad recipe following.

For the salad, mix together the fresh arugula, half of the apples, and the bacon. In a small pan, cook the chopped yellow onion in 1 tablespoon of the oil with salt and pepper. Cook until caramelized. Transfer to the salad and toss thoroughly. In another sauce pan, cook the remaining apples on medium heat. Stir in the apple cider vinegar, 1 tablespoon of oil, brown sugar, salt, and pepper. Cook on low heat until the apples are almost fully cooked. Stir with the rest of the salad. Dress the salad with the prepared dressing, using the amount of your liking. Serve immediately after dressing.

Chicken Chopped Salad

2 grilled chicken breasts, cut into medium cubes
1 head living lettuce
1 Granny Smith apple, chopped into cubes
½ pound small fingerling potatoes, cut into halves

FOR THE DRESSING:
3 pieces of crispy bacon, plus extra to use as salad
    topping (chopped or crushed in food processor)
½ cup maple syrup
½ cup olive oil
Zest of 1 orange
Salt
Pepper

Preheat oven to 450°.

Prepare the vinaigrette — combine bacon, maple
syrup, olive oil, orange zest, salt and pepper in a
bowl and stir until mixed thoroughly. Set aside.

On a medium sheet pan lined with foil, spread
the potatoes out, flat side down. Drizzle with 1
tablespoon of the dressing, and sprinkle with salt
and pepper. Bake in a preheated 450 degree oven
until crispy and golden brown, or until you can poke
with a fork (35 to 45 minutes).

Meanwhile, in a large bowl, toss together the
lettuce, chopped apple and grilled chicken. When the
potatoes are done, cool for about 10 minutes, then
transfer into the lettuce. Dress with desired amount
of the dressing. Sprinkle with remaining bacon and
serve immediately.

Spicy Shrimp Salad

½ pound shrimp, peeled and deveined
4-6 cups arugula
4 cloves garlic, minced
2 tablespoons capers
1 cup olive oil
Juice of 1 lemon
1 teaspoon red pepper flakes
½ cup fresh mango, cubed
Salt (as needed)
Freshly ground black pepper (as needed)

Sauté the shrimp in ¼ cup of olive oil, two of the minced garlic cloves, 1 teaspoon of lemon juice, salt, freshly ground black pepper, and a pinch of the red pepper flakes. Sauté the shrimp on medium-high heat 3 minutes per side or until chewy and pink. Remove from heat, cover, and set aside for later.

For the dressing, mix the remaining olive oil, lemon juice, minced garlic, red pepper flakes, salt, and black pepper with the capers in a small bowl. Set aside.

In a big bowl, mix the shrimp with the arugula (make sure to use the oil leftover from cooking the shrimp) and the mango. Toss in the dressing and finish off with some more salt and pepper. Serve immediately at room temperature.

Sweet & Spicy Arugula Salad

2 avocados, peeled and diced
4-6 cups arugula
2 heirloom tomatoes, diced
¼ red onion, chopped roughly
2 fresh peaches, diced

FOR THE DRESSING:
¾ cup olive oil
Juice of 1 lemon
Zest of 1 lemon
2 teaspoons Dijon mustard
3 basil leaves, minced
1 teaspoon red pepper flakes
2 garlic cloves, minced
1 teaspoon honey
Salt
Pepper

Whisk together the olive oil, lemon juice, lemon zest, Dijon mustard, basil, red pepper flakes, garlic, honey, salt, and pepper in a small bowl. Set aside.

In a large bowl, combine the arugula, avocados, tomatoes, onions, and peaches. Dress with the prepared dressing. Serve at room temperature or chilled.

Summer Pasta Salad

(v)

1 yellow bell pepper, diced into cubes
1 large red onion, roughly chopped
2 heads broccoli, chopped into pieces
½ box shell pasta, cooked according to package directions
4 ears fresh corn (or 4 cups of frozen corn)
Your favorite French vinaigrette for the sauce

Stir everything together in a big bowl, and serve at room temperature with the vinaigrette.

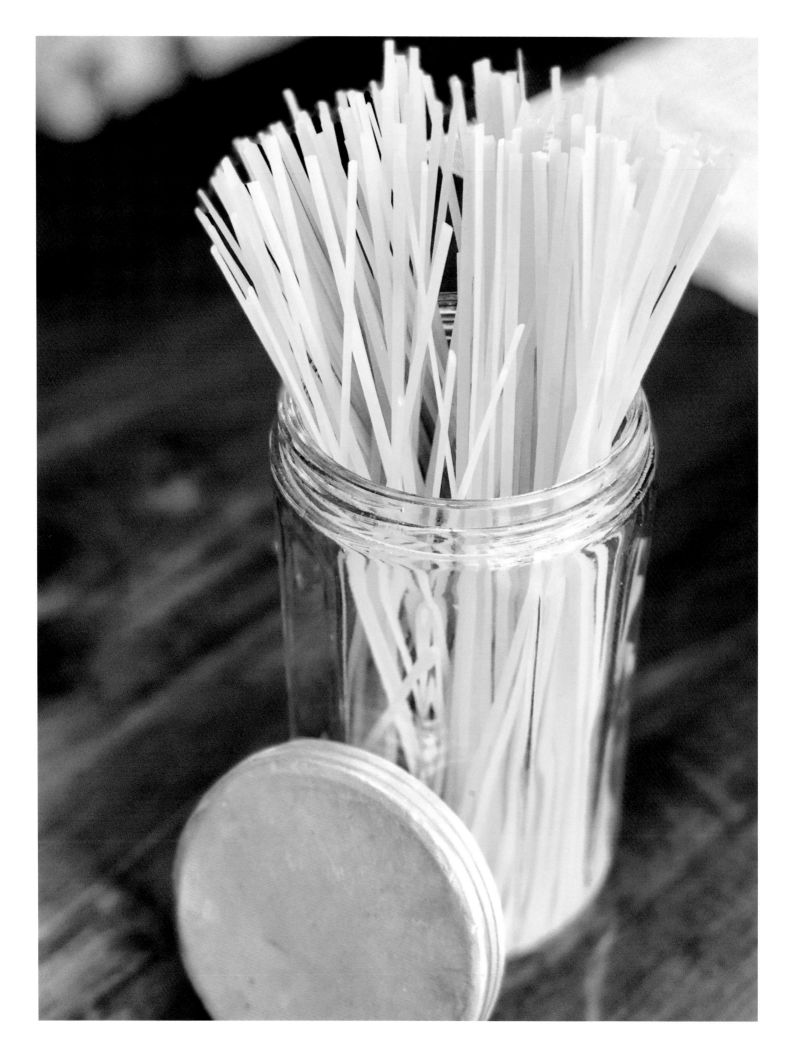

Chicken Noodle Soup with a Twist

4 cups chicken stock
1 box spaghetti
6 large carrots, peeled and cut into circles
3 large celery stocks, cut into pieces
1 large yellow onion, diced
1 cup chopped baby portobello mushrooms
4 tablespoons olive oil
3 cloves garlic, minced
1 tablespoon dairy-free butter
2 sprigs thyme leaves
Salt
Pepper

In a large stock pot, heat the 4 tablespoons of olive oil on medium-high heat. Once heated, add diced onion, carrots, and celery. Cook on medium heat for 15 to 20 minutes, or until the vegetables are almost fully cooked. Then, add the chopped mushrooms and cook for 5 more minutes. And the garlic and stir constantly for 30 seconds. Add the chicken stock next, bring to a large boil, then add the spaghetti. Cook the pasta soup for 10 minutes, or until the pasta is fully cooked. Add the thyme leaves, butter, salt, and pepper. Cook for another 10 minutes on simmer. Serve with warm bread or croutons. Chill leftovers in the fridge.

Creamy Potato Fennel Soup

1 pound Yukon gold potatoes, quartered
½ fennel bulb, roughly chopped
2 yellow onions, roughly chopped
4 cups chicken stock
Olive oil (as needed)
Salt and pepper
1 garlic clove, roughly chopped (or ½ teaspoon garlic powder)
2 tablespoons chives (for garnish)
Croutons (for garnish)
Bacon crumbles (for garnish)

Sauté the onions and fennel in olive oil until soft. Meanwhile chop the potatoes (skins on) and boil them separately in a large pot until cooked through and skins fall off. Remove from heat and drain. Remove skins. Add onion mixture into the pot with the potatoes.

Add chicken stock and bring to a boil. Turn off heat and blend soup with a hand held blender until smooth. Add salt and pepper to taste. Drizzle a little olive oil on individual soup bowls. Serve hot. Garnish with chives, bacon, and croutons.

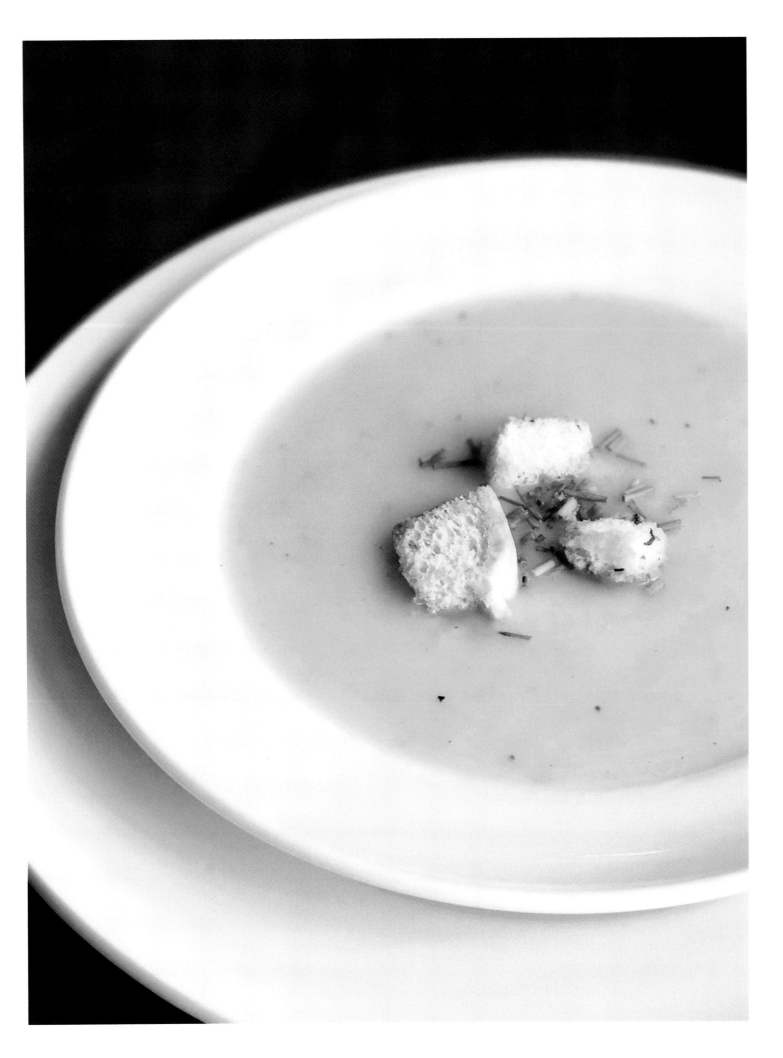

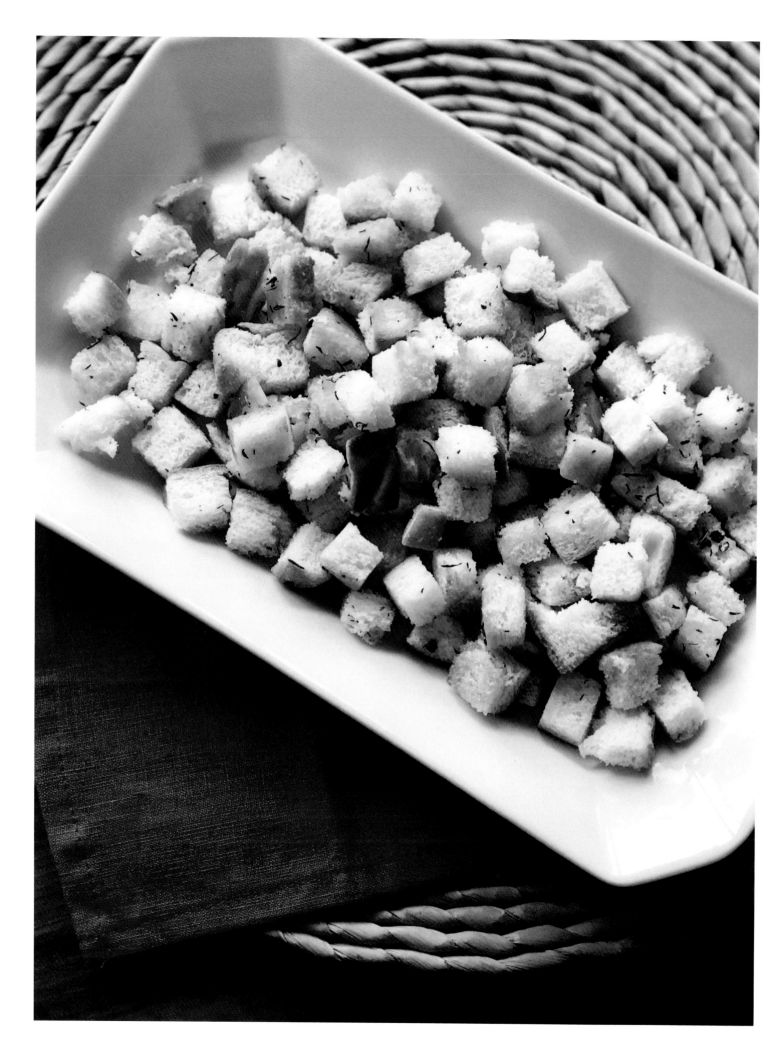

Crunchy Thyme Croutons

2 cups cubed bread
2 tablespoons olive oil
Salt and freshly ground black pepper, to taste
Dried thyme, to taste

Preheat oven to 350°.

Cut the bread into small cubes. Place on sheet pan in a single layer. Toss with olive oil. Sprinkle with the seasonings. Bake at 350 degrees for 10 to 15 minutes or until golden and crisp. Serve warm as an appetizer or with soup.

Cauliflower Leek Soup

2 heads cauliflower
1 leek
8 cups chicken stock
1 bay leaf
2 garlic cloves
3 tablespoons olive oil
1 medium yellow onion
1 teaspoon fresh or dried thyme
Salt
Pepper

Cut the cauliflower into bite sized pieces, mince the garlic, cut the leek into circles, mince the thyme (if using fresh), and chop the onion. Meanwhile, in a large stock pot, heat the oil on medium heat until sizzling. Add the onions and leeks, and cook until caramelized. Add the chopped cauliflower and garlic, stir constantly for 2 minutes. Stir in the chicken stock, bay leaf, thyme, salt, and pepper. Bring to a large boil, and then turn down to simmer. With an immersion blender, blend the soup, keeping the head of the blender submerged in the soup. Blend until smooth. Cook on low heat for 5 more minutes. Serve warm with croutons (recipe on page 47).

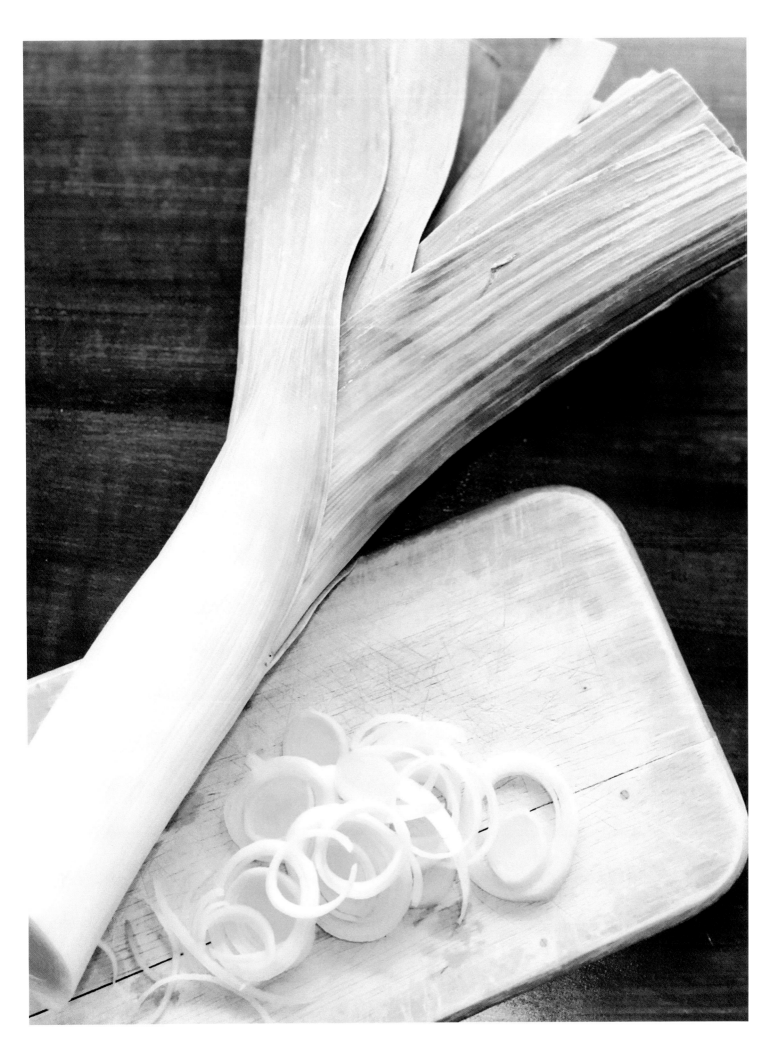

Sides

Parmesan Roasted Zucchini Strips

2 large zucchini, cut lengthwise into ¼ inch thick strips
1 cup panko breadcrumbs
¼ cup dairy-free parmesan cheese
Olive oil
Salt
Pepper

Preheat oven to 400°.

Combine the breadcrumbs, cheese, drizzle of olive oil and salt and pepper.

In one layer arrange the zucchini slices on a sheet pan lined with foil. Drizzle with olive oil and the breadcrumb and cheese mixture. Bake for 15 to 20 minutes or until cooked and the topping is lightly brown. Serve warm.

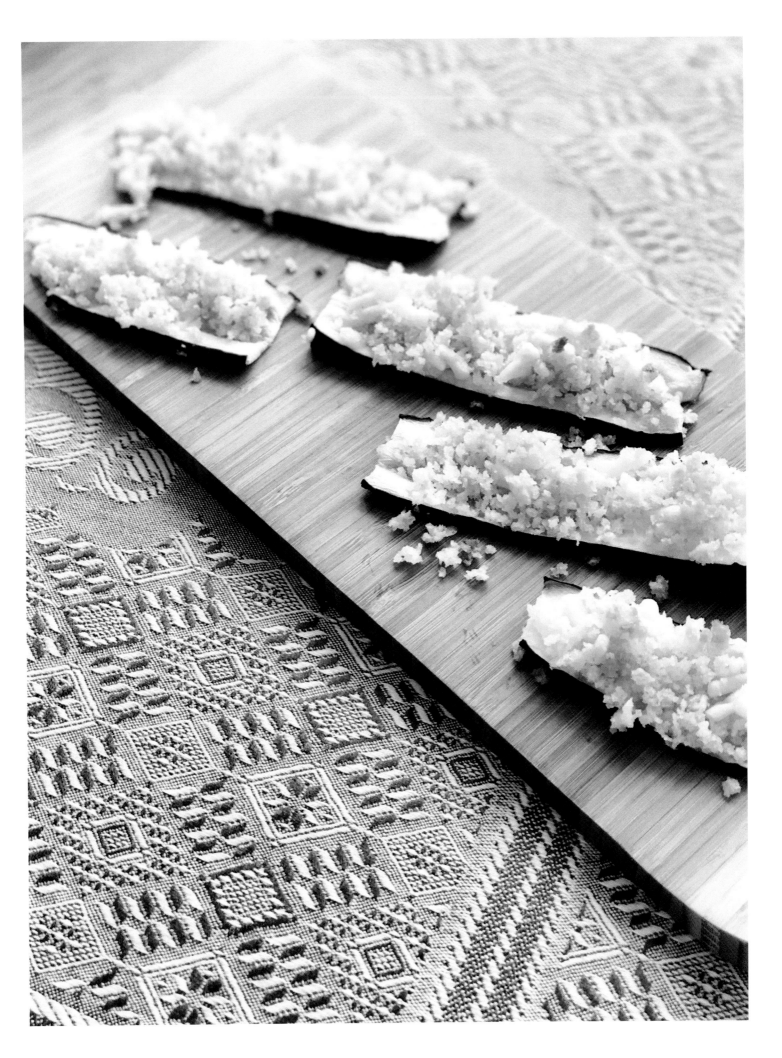

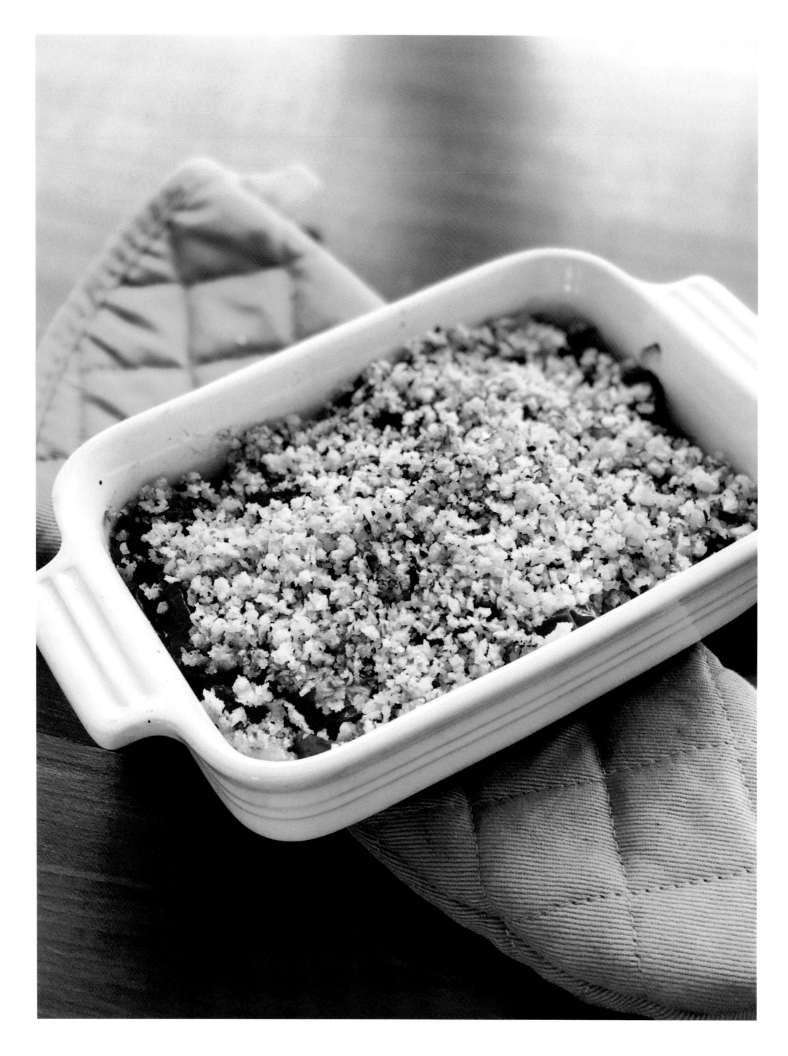

Cherry Tomato Gratin

(v)

1 pint red cherry tomatoes
¼ cup olive oil
½ cup breadcrumbs
¼ teaspoon cumin
½ teaspoon oregano
1 garlic clove, minced
Salt (to taste)
Freshly ground black pepper (to taste)
Sugar (for sprinkling)

Preheat oven to 400°.

Chop the cherry tomatoes in half and transfer to a small oven proof baking dish. Drizzle with half of the olive oil and set aside.

Combine the breadcrumbs, cumin, garlic powder, oregano, salt, pepper and the rest of the olive oil in a medium sized bowl. Sprinkle all of the breadcrumbs on top of the tomatoes. Bake for 20 to 25 minutes or until the breadcrumbs are golden brown. Serve warm.

Cumin Cauliflower

2½ tablespoons dairy-free butter
2 tablespoons olive oil
2 cups small chopped cauliflower
2 teaspoons ground cumin
Salt (to taste)
Freshly ground black pepper (to taste)
2 tablespoons water

Cook the cauliflower in a medium sauté pan with the butter, olive oil, salt, pepper and cumin on medium heat until cooked thoroughly, about 22 minutes. Occasionally pour a little of the water in the pan to steam the cauliflower. Cover with a lid after putting the water in the pan. When the cauliflower is done, add 1 teaspoon of butter and a little sprinkle of cumin. Combine and serve warm.

Balsamic Onions

3 tablespoons olive oil
1 white onion, chopped into rings
¼-⅓ cup balsamic vinegar (it depends on how strong you want the flavor)
Salt
Freshly ground black pepper

Sauté onions in pan for 5 minutes until partially cooked. Then slowly add half of the balsamic vinegar stirring constantly. Put pan lid on and let cook for 5 more minutes. Remove the lid and add the rest of the balsamic vinegar. Cook with NO lid for 3 more minutes, and transfer into a bowl. Serve hot with salt and pepper to taste on top.

Pan Roasted Garlic Potatoes

10 Yukon gold potatoes
10 red skin potatoes
Olive oil (as needed)
1 small onion, roughly chopped
1 teaspoon dried thyme
1 teaspoon dried oregano
2 teaspoons minced garlic
¼ teaspoon salt
½ teaspoon freshly ground black pepper

Cut the potatoes into pencil width circles. Heat the olive oil in a pan at medium heat. Add the chopped onion and let cook until lightly caramelized. Slowly add the potatoes, and let them cook for 10 to 15 minutes (making sure to scrape the pan often). Add spices, garlic, more oil, cover until fully cooked (checking them often.) Serve warm.

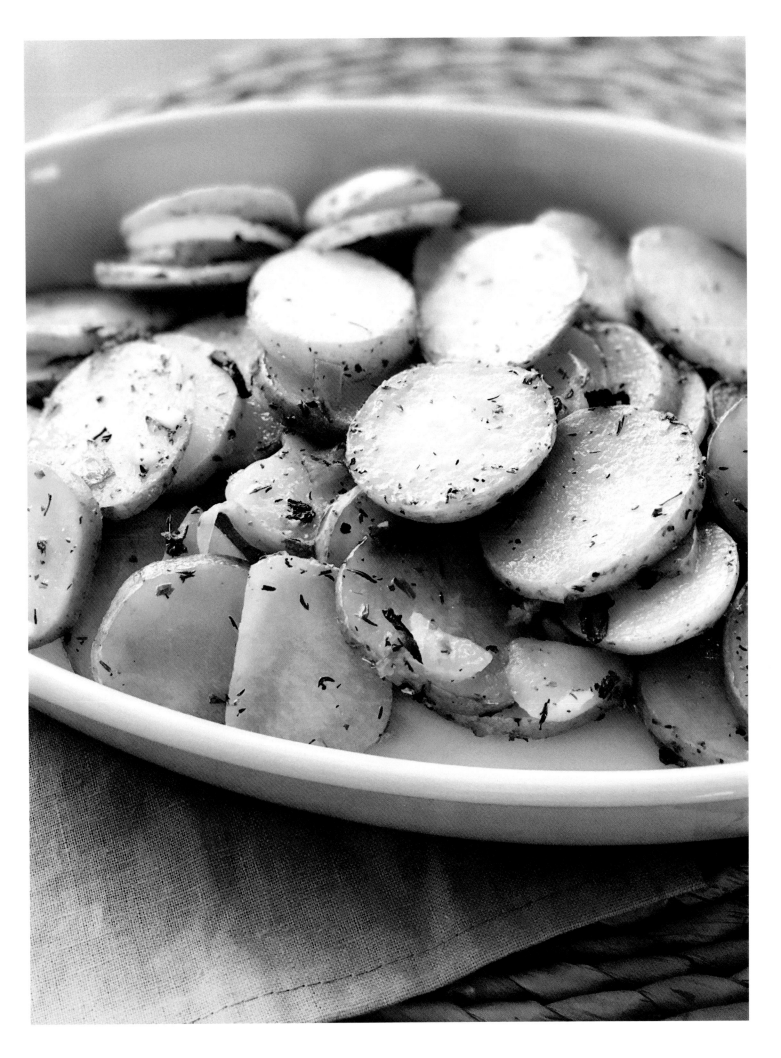

Roasted Garlic Mashed Potatoes

5 Idaho potatoes, peeled and chopped into chunks
Dairy-free butter (as needed)
Dairy-free milk (as needed)
3 garlic cloves, roasted
Salt
Freshly ground black pepper

Preheat oven to 400°.

Take the garlic cloves and wrap them in foil with a drizzle of olive oil in it. Cook in the oven until colored and soft. Then smash it to create a paste. Set aside.

Boil potatoes in water in a large pot for 40 to 45 minutes. Mash potatoes with butter, milk and garlic paste, salt, and pepper. Serve hot.

Roasted Green Pepper Rice

2 green bell peppers, cut into thick slices
1 inch of a jalapeño
Zest and juice of 1 lime
¼ cup cilantro
2 tablespoons cooked white or yellow onions
Salt and pepper
Olive oil
2 cups uncooked long grain rice (cooked according to package directions)

Preheat oven to 425°.

On a sheet pan lined with foil lay out the bell peppers evenly and drizzle with olive oil and salt and pepper.

Roast peppers in a preheated oven for 20 to 25 minutes or until lightly charred and soft.

In a food processor add the cooked peppers with the leftover oil from the pan, jalapeño, lime zest and juice, onions, cilantro, and more salt and pepper to taste. Pulse until finely chopped. Combine the green pepper mixture with the cooked rice and serve hot or at room temperature.

Salsa Rice

3 cups Basmati rice (cooked according to package directions)
3 pints red tomatoes, chopped roughly
1 yellow onion, chopped roughly
Dried oregano
Pinch of salt
Freshly ground black pepper
3 tablespoons olive oil
1 teaspoon chili powder
¼ to ⅛ teaspoon of coriander
⅛ teaspoon cumin
5 basil leaves, chopped roughly

Sauté the onions with the olive oil in a large pan until lightly browned. Add the tomatoes to the onions and then sprinkle the oregano, salt, chili powder, coriander, cumin, and pepper into it. Let it simmer covered until the tomato juice comes out. Pour onto the cooked rice and serve hot with basil as garnish.

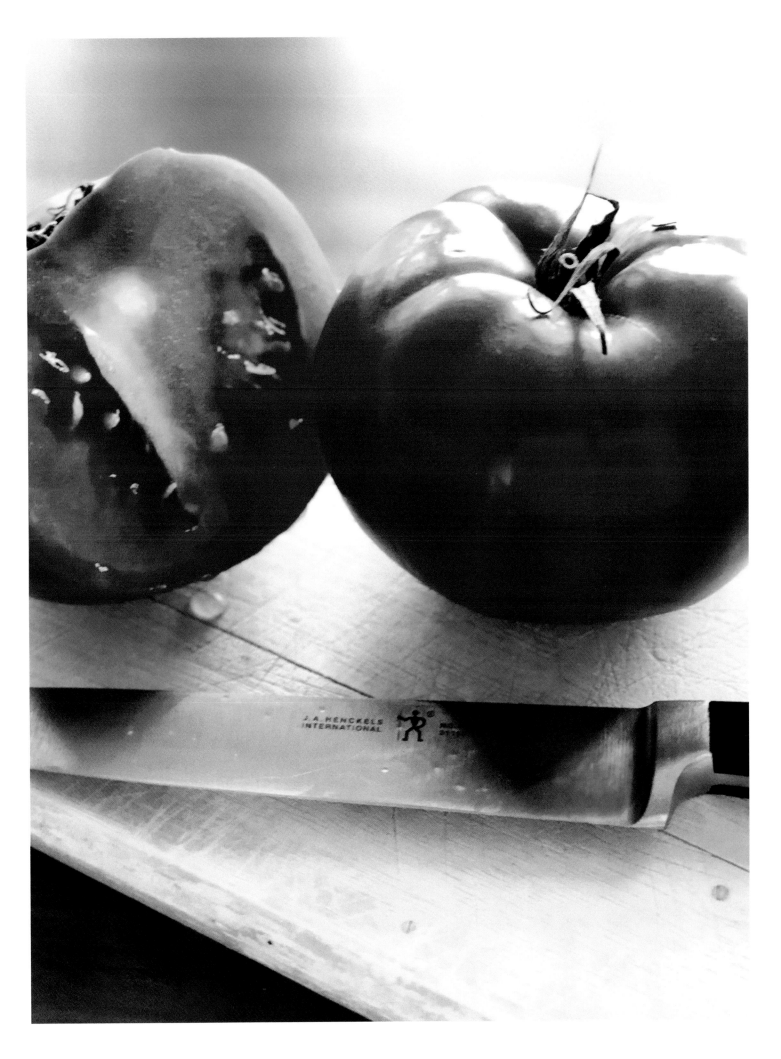

Smoky Spiced Rice

3 cups long grain white rice (cooked according to package directions in low salt chicken stock)
1 teaspoon paprika
2 tablespoons olive oil
Salt
½ red jalapeño
¼ teaspoon coriander
Freshly ground black pepper

Roast the jalapeño over an open flame until charred. Once very charred, pull off the stove and remove the black parts. Chop them up into small strips. Set aside.

Put everything into a pot, and stir. Heat the stove up on medium-high, until boiling. Turn the heat down to medium, and cook for 15 more minutes or until fluffy. Serve warm. Add the jalapeño to the rice with the coriander, oil, pepper, and paprika. Serve warm.

Fried Rice with Ginger Sauce

Canola oil

1 zucchini, chopped into thin slices

5 medium sized carrots, sliced thinly

2 heads broccoli, roughly chopped

1 yellow onion, roughly chopped

½ pound green beans,
   chopped into half inch pieces

2 cups cooked Basmati rice
   (cooked according to package directions)

3 shoshito peppers, cut in strips

FOR THE SAUCE:

1½ cups soy sauce

4-5 tablespoons honey

2 tablespoons water mixed with 2 teaspoons
   cornstarch (use 1 tablespoon of mixture)

2 teaspoons grated ginger

1 teaspoon sesame seeds (optional)

Put the soy sauce in a saucepan with the honey and lemon juice. Slowly add the water and cornstarch mixture. Then add the grated ginger last. Serve warm on top of the stir fry.

Cut all the vegetables. Cook the onions in a pan with canola oil, until lightly caramelized. Then slowly add the green beans then carrots then zucchini and broccoli (all two minutes apart.) Cook the vegetables until bright and juicy (don't over cook). Cook rice. Add cooked rice to the vegetables. Drizzle the sauce on top. Serve hot.

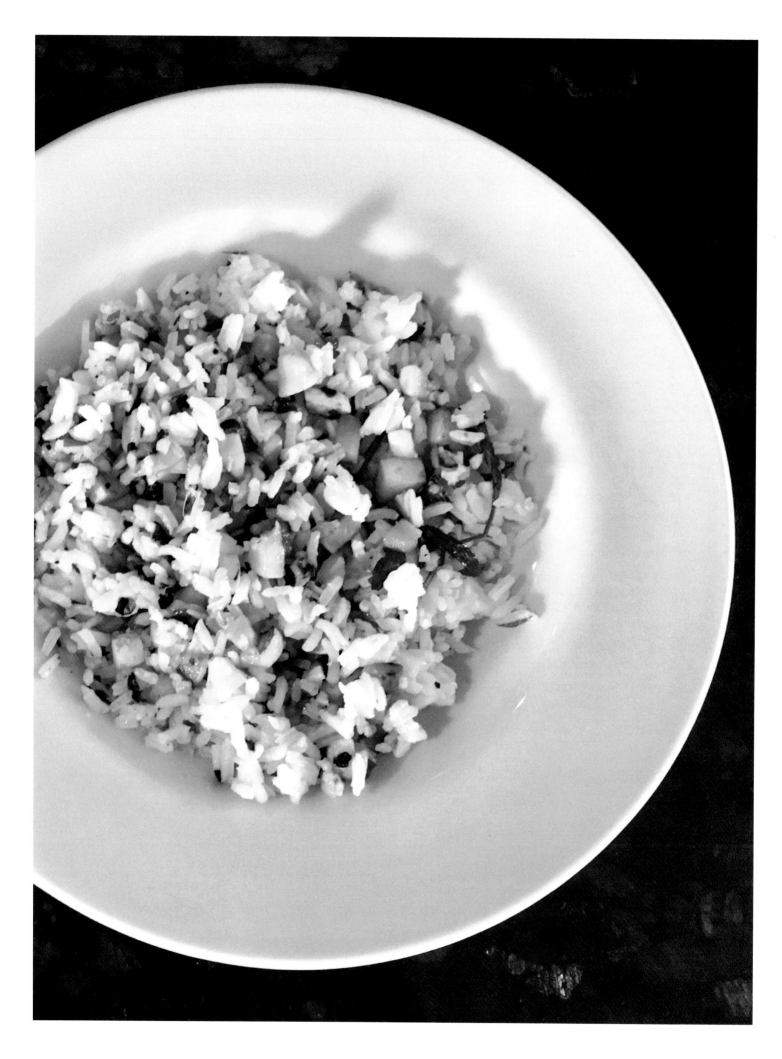

Summer Squash Fried Rice

2½ cups precooked Basmati rice
2 medium yellow summer squash, cut into small cubes
1 shallot, minced
1 garlic clove, minced
1 handful chopped fresh parsley
2 tablespoons dairy-free butter
1 tablespoon olive oil
Salt and pepper

In a medium sauté pan cook the shallots with 1 tablespoon of the butter and olive oil until lightly caramelized. Add the summer squash and cook until squash is soft and lightly brown. Add the garlic and parsley and cook for 1 more minute. Add the remaining 1 tablespoon of butter and salt and pepper.

Add the cooked rice to the pan with the squash. Stir together and serve hot.

Sweet Summertime Slaw

1 head iceberg lettuce, shredded
1 head radicchio, shredded
2 carrots, shredded
3 tablespoons capers
2 ears fresh corn, boiled and cut off the cob

FOR THE DRESSING:
Juice of 1 lemon
Juice of 1 orange
Zest of 1 lime
Fresh chives, minced
½ cup olive oil
2 tablespoons Dijon mustard
1 teaspoon whole grain Dijon mustard
Salt and pepper, to taste

In a large bowl, toss the lettuce, radicchio, carrots, capers and corn together. Set aside. In a small bowl, whisk together the lemon juice, orange juice, lime zest, fresh chives, olive oil, Dijon mustards, salt and pepper. Pour the dressing into the lettuce bowl and toss gently. Serve cold or at room temperature as a side dish.

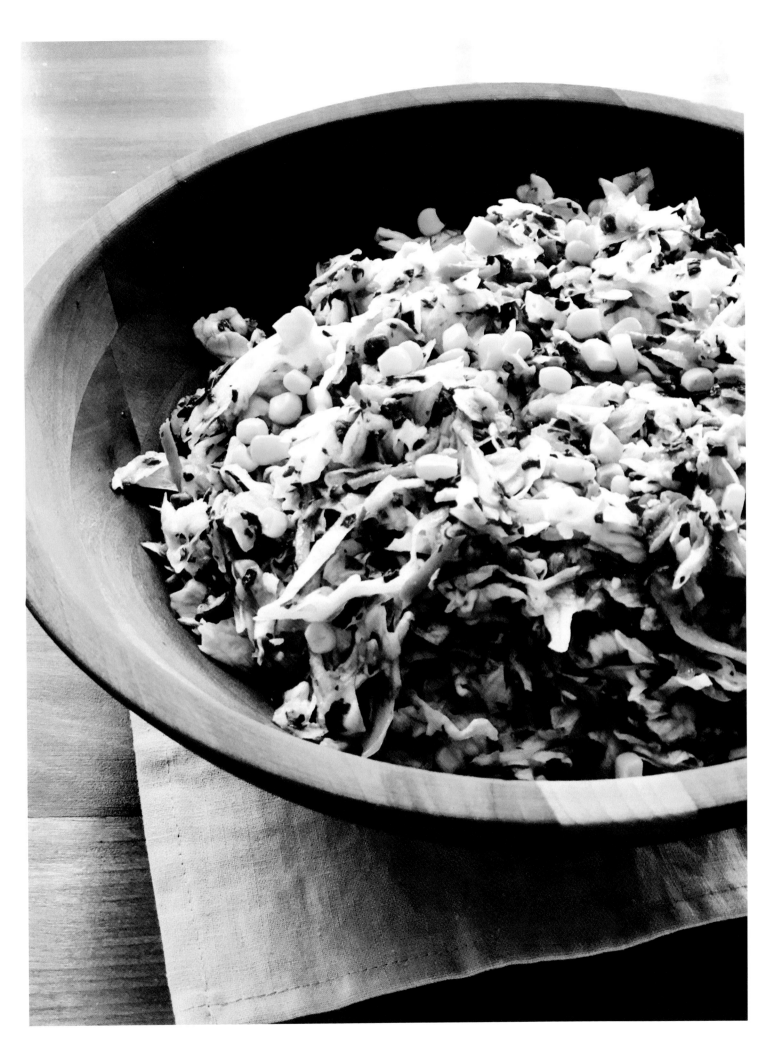

Main Courses

Easiest Tomato Sauce

2 cans crushed tomatoes (28 ounce each)
½ teaspoon dried oregano
1 large yellow onion, finely chopped
3 medium garlic cloves, minced
¼ teaspoon dried chili flakes
2 tablespoons olive oil
Salt
Pepper

In a medium stock pot, cook the onion in the oil with salt and pepper. After the onions become slightly browned, add the garlic. Pour in the crushed tomatoes and stir. Add the oregano, chili flakes, salt, and pepper. You can use this in the lasagna, on pasta, pizza, etc. Chill until used.

Spinach Pesto Pasta

½ box linguine pasta (cooked according to package directions)
1 clove garlic, minced
Dairy-free parmesan cheese (optional)

FOR THE SAUCE:
6 ounces fresh spinach
Salt
Pepper
2 tablespoons water
1 tablespoon olive oil
3 tablespoons freshly squeezed lemon juice

Cook the spinach in the olive oil until wilts. Transfer the spinach and oil into a blender, and add the salt, pepper, lemon juice, and water. (Make sure to cover the blender with a kitchen towel, as the liquid will be very hot). Blend it until smooth, and set aside until later.

Toss together with the garlic and pasta and serve at room temperature. Sprinkle with dairy-free parmesan cheese.

Lemon Garlic Linguine

½ box linguine pasta (cooked according to package directions)
2 zucchini, cut into thin circles
¼ cup plus 1 teaspoon olive oil
1 small yellow onion, finely chopped
1 garlic clove, minced
¼ teaspoon dairy-free butter
Zest of 1 lemon
Juice of ½ lemon
2 large basil leaves, minced
Salt and freshly ground pepper (to taste)

Sauté the garlic and onions in a stockpot with ¼ cup olive oil until lightly caramelized. Add the zucchini slices and cook until almost transparent (or done to your liking). Add the cooked pasta to the zucchini and onion mixture and toss together with the lemon zest, lemon juice, basil, salt, pepper, butter, and remaining 1 teaspoon olive oil.

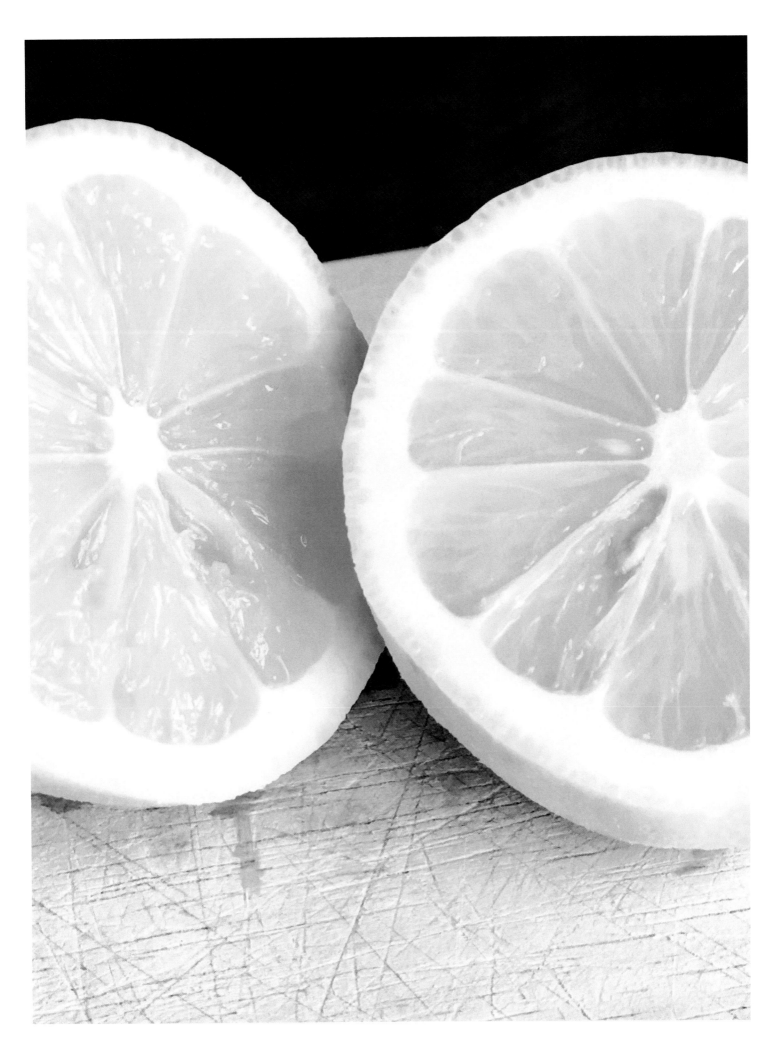

Hearty Vegetable Lasagna

9-12 sheets of uncooked, dried vegan lasagna noodles
3 cups tomato sauce (see recipe on page 72)
2 cups dairy-free shredded mozzarella
3 zucchini, sliced in thin circles
1 package small baby mushrooms, sliced
1½-2 cups panko bread crumbs
6-10 tablespoons olive oil
Salt
Pepper
1-2 teaspoons dried oregano
½ teaspoon dried chili flakes
1 package frozen spinach
2 small yellow onions, chopped

Preheat oven to 425°.

Bring a large pot of salted water to boil. Place the noodles in the water one by one and cook until one minute over al dente.

Meanwhile, place cut zucchini in a medium sauté pan with 2 tablespoons of olive oil. Cook the zucchini until caramelized or translucent.

In a separate small sauté pan, cook the baby mushrooms and 1 tablespoon of olive oil until tender.

In a large sauté pan, cook the spinach with the chopped yellow onions and 2 tablespoons of olive oil, salt, and pepper.

Cook the spinach until defrosted. In a small bowl, mix together the breadcrumbs, 3 tablespoons of olive oil, salt, pepper, chili flakes, and oregano.

Now assemble the lasagna. In a medium casserole dish, make a thin layer of the tomato sauce on the bottom, and place three cooked lasagna noodles lengthwise on top of the sauce. Spread some of the spinach mixture on top of each lasagna noodle. Add ½ of the shredded dairy-free cheese. Add a few more spoonfuls of the sauce. Place some of the zucchini and mushrooms on top of the spinach and sauce. Place three more lasagna noodles on top of that. Repeat these steps until you reach the top of the casserole dish. Finally on the top sprinkle the remaining dairy-free shredded mozzarella and pat the breadcrumbs in an even layer.

Bake the lasagna in a 425 degree oven for 10 to 20 minutes or until the breadcrumbs are golden brown. Serve warm. This dish is great if you freeze it or if you have it leftover for days.

Grilled Citrus Salmon with Cauliflower Leek Couscous

Zest and juice of 2 lemons
Zest and juice of 2 oranges
2 garlic cloves
2 teaspoons fresh thyme
1 tablespoon olive oil
4 salmon fillets

FOR THE COUSCOUS:
1 tablespoon freshly squeezed orange juice
1 cup chicken stock
¾ cup uncooked couscous
½ leek, cut in circles
1 shallot, minced
3 spoonfuls salmon marinade
1 small head of cauliflower
1 garlic clove
1½ teaspoons dairy-free butter
2 tablespoons olive oil
Salt
Pepper

Preheat oven to 400°.

Boil the chicken stock with 1 tablespoon of the olive oil, orange juice, salt, and pepper. Once it boils stir in the couscous and turn off the heat.
In a small pot, steam cauliflower until tender. In a medium sauté pan, sauté the garlic, leeks, shallots, and steamed cauliflower in the butter and rest of the olive oil. Sprinkle with salt and pepper. Cook for about 5 to 10 minutes. Combine the couscous with the cauliflower mix. Serve warm with the salmon.

Whisk together the juice and zest of the lemons and oranges, garlic, thyme, oil, salt, and pepper. Place the salmon in the marinade, cover with plastic wrap, and chill in a fridge for at least 30 minutes, letting the juices and flavors soak into the salmon. After the salmon marinates, heat a medium cast iron skillet on medium-high heat. Place salmon in the heated skillet. Cook for 4 minutes on each side until you have a good sear. Transfer the skillet to a preheated oven at 400 degrees for 5 more minutes. Serve with the couscous.

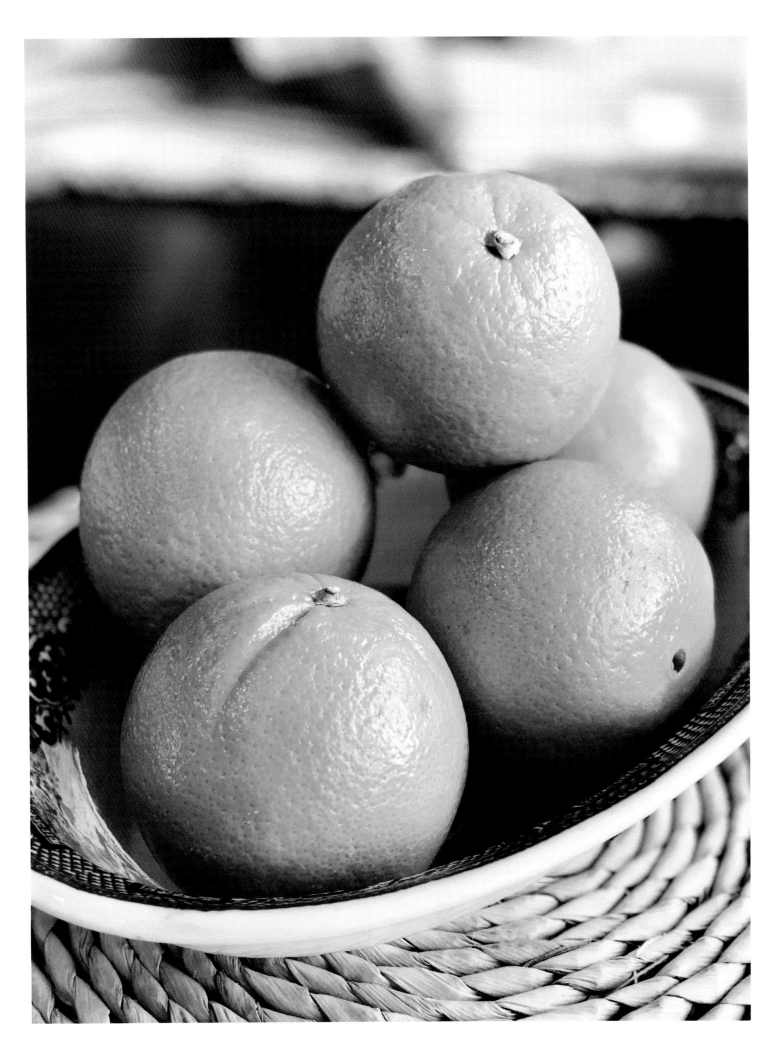

Lemon Garlic Grilled Salmon with Basil Peach Sauce & Spinach Pesto

4 salmon fillets
¾ cup olive oil
Zest and juice of 1 lemon
2 teaspoons Dijon mustard
3 basil leaves, minced
1 teaspoon red pepper flakes
2 garlic cloves, minced
1 teaspoon honey
Salt
Pepper

FOR THE SAUCE:
4 fresh peaches, peeled and chopped
1 tablespoon honey
4 tablespoons water
½ teaspoon chili powder
4 basil leaves
2 tablespoons fresh chives

FOR THE PESTO:
2 cups fresh spinach
10 fresh basil leaves
A handful of fresh parsley
⅓ cup olive oil
Juice of 1 lemon
Zest of 1 lemon
2 tablespoons fresh chives
Salt
Pepper

Preheat oven to 375°.

Whisk everything together in a large bowl. Place the salmon in the marinade bowl, cover with plastic wrap and put in the fridge, marinate for one hour.

Heat a grill on medium heat. Place the salmon skin side down on the grill. Grill for 5 minutes on each side. Transfer to the oven and bake for 10 more minutes until the salmon is flaky and cooked fully. Serve with the pesto and peach sauce.

For the sauce: sauté the peaches with the honey and water on medium heat until bubbling. Transfer to a blender, add chili powder, chives, and basil and blend until smooth. Serve at room temperature.

For the pesto: transfer into a food processor and pulse until chunky and combined. Serve on top of salmon.

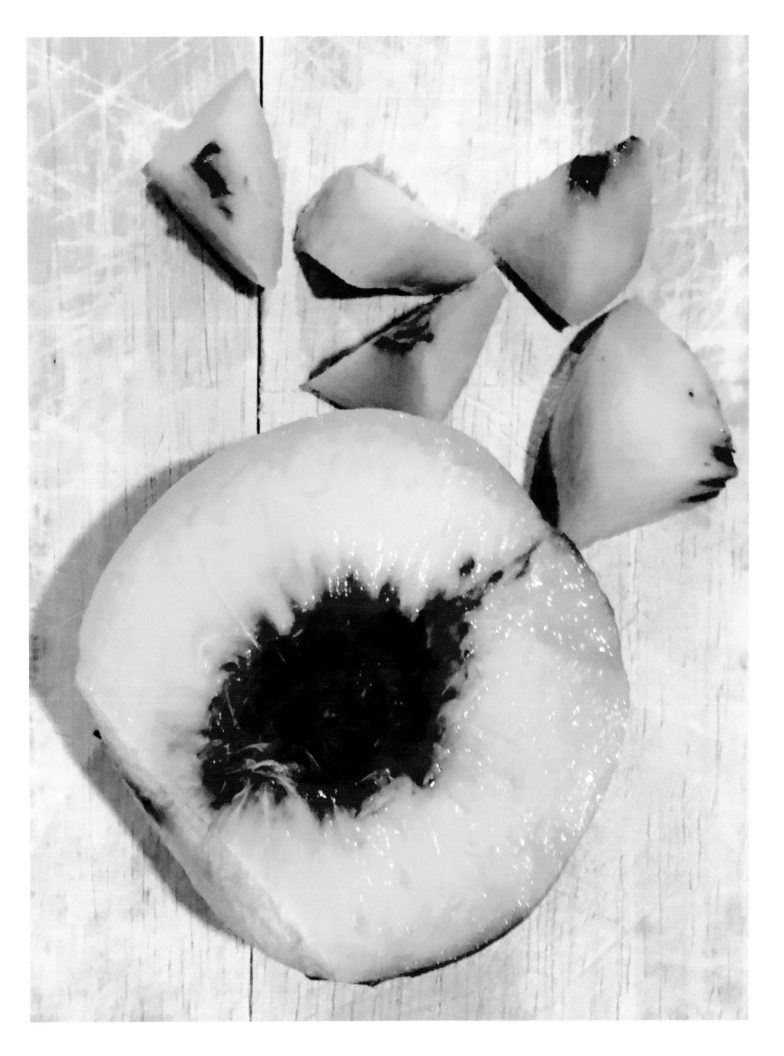

Light Onion Parsley Rice with Scallops

2 cups Basmati rice (cooked according to package directions)
1 large onion, chopped finely
Olive oil
1 tablespoon dairy-free butter
2 tablespoons white wine
Fresh parsley, finely chopped
1 pound sea scallops
½ cup all purpose flour

Cook the onions in a pan with the oil until lightly browned. Add the wine and let cook down for at least 10 minutes. Add the sauce to the cooked rice and add the chopped parsley. Fold in the butter. Serve warm.

For the scallops, get a large sauté pan heated on medium heat with 1 tablespoon olive oil. Dredge the scallops in the flour brushing off the extra. Place them in the heated pan to get a good sear. Turn after 2 minutes of cooking on one side and cook for 3 more minutes on the other. Serve immediately with the rice.

Shrimp with Cauliflower Purée

FOR THE CAULIFLOWER PURÉE:

1 head cauliflower, cut into small pieces, steamed
   and drained
1 tablespoon olive oil
½ teaspoon paprika
¼ teaspoon cumin
1 teaspoon fresh parsley, minced
Pinch of cayenne pepper
Pinch of salt and cracked pepper

FOR THE SHRIMP RUB:

25 shrimp
3 teaspoons paprika
1½ teaspoons cumin
¼ teaspoon of chili powder
Salt and pepper

Make the puree: blend together in blender or food
processor until smooth. Sprinkle with cumin on top
and set aside to serve with shrimp.

Wash and dry peeled and deveined shrimp. Coat
shrimp with olive oil and then roll in rub.

Cook shrimp in an oiled skillet for 6 minutes, flip
half-way through. Cook until shrimp are pink.

Serve warm with dip on side.

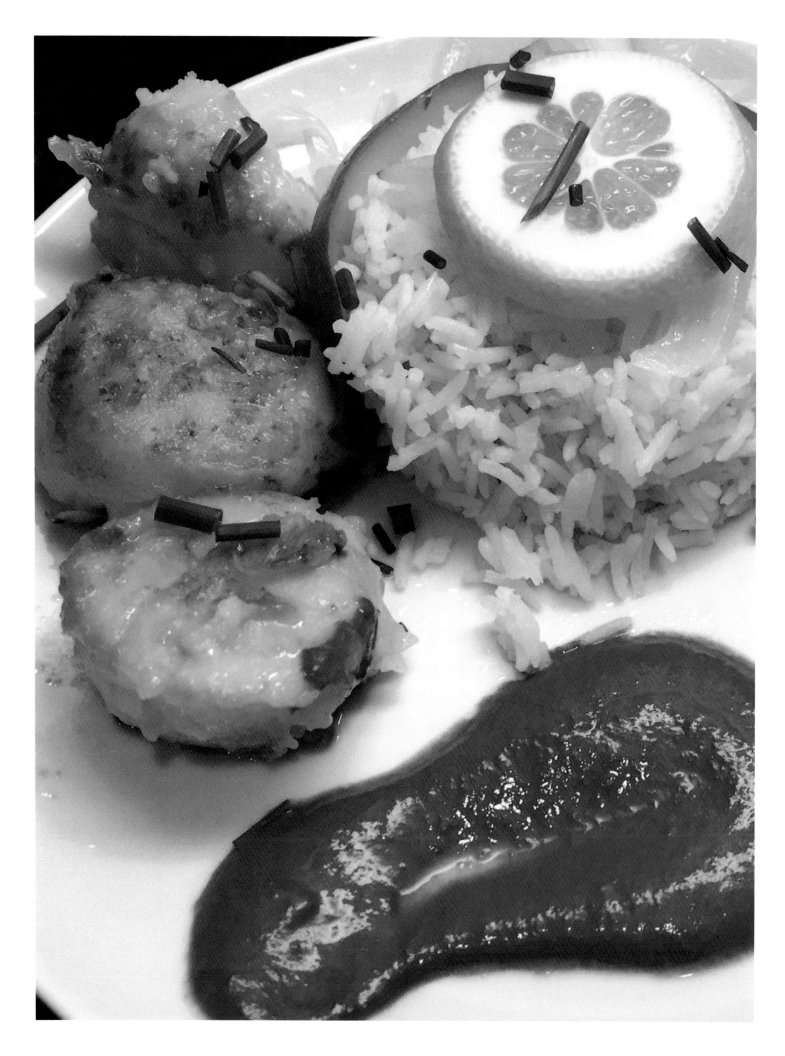

Sea Scallops with Spinach Sauce

FOR THE SCALLOPS:

1 dozen fresh sea scallops

2 tablespoons all purpose flour

1 yellow onion, roughly chopped

3 tablespoons olive oil

3 cups white rice (cooked according to package directions)

1 tablespoon white wine

FOR THE SAUCE:

6 ounces fresh spinach

Salt

Pepper

2 tablespoons water

1 tablespoon olive oil

3 tablespoons freshly squeezed lemon juice

Cook the spinach in the olive oil until it wilts. Transfer the spinach and oil into a blender, and add the salt, pepper, lemon juice, and water. (Make sure to cover the blender with a kitchen towel, as the liquid will be very hot). Blend until smooth, and set aside until later.

Sauté the onions in the white wine and olive oil until lightly caramelized. Dredge the scallops in the flour and sear in the pan of onions. Cook the scallops for 3 minutes on each side so they have a golden sear and juicy insides. Serve immediately with the sauce.

Garlic Shrimp with Vegetable Pasta

FOR THE SHRIMP:
1 clove garlic, minced
Salt
Pinch of paprika
Freshly ground black pepper
Zest and juice of 1 lemon
4 tablespoons olive oil
10 large shrimp, peeled, deveined, and tails removed

FOR THE PASTA:
½ pound uncooked spaghetti
1 clove garlic, minced
Salt and freshly ground black pepper, to taste
1 zucchini, cut into circles
1 yellow onion, roughly chopped
1 heirloom tomato, diced
2 ears fresh corn
Olive oil, as needed

Mix the garlic, 3 tablespoons of oil, lemon, salt, pepper, and paprika together and set aside. Place the shrimp in the bowl with the garlic oil mixture. Heat a large pan on medium with the remaining oil. Place the shrimp in the hot pan and cook for 6 minutes (3 minutes per side) or until pink and chewy. Set aside to serve with pasta. Serve warm.

Cook the pasta according to the package. Set aside. Boil the corn in a pot of water for about 10 minutes. Next, cut the corn off of the cob and set aside. Sauté the zucchini in a pan of olive oil on medium heat until almost transparent and set aside. Cook the onions in a pan of olive oil on medium heat until lightly caramelized, and set aside. Dice the tomato and set aside. Toss everything together in a big bowl with the shrimp. Serve warm.

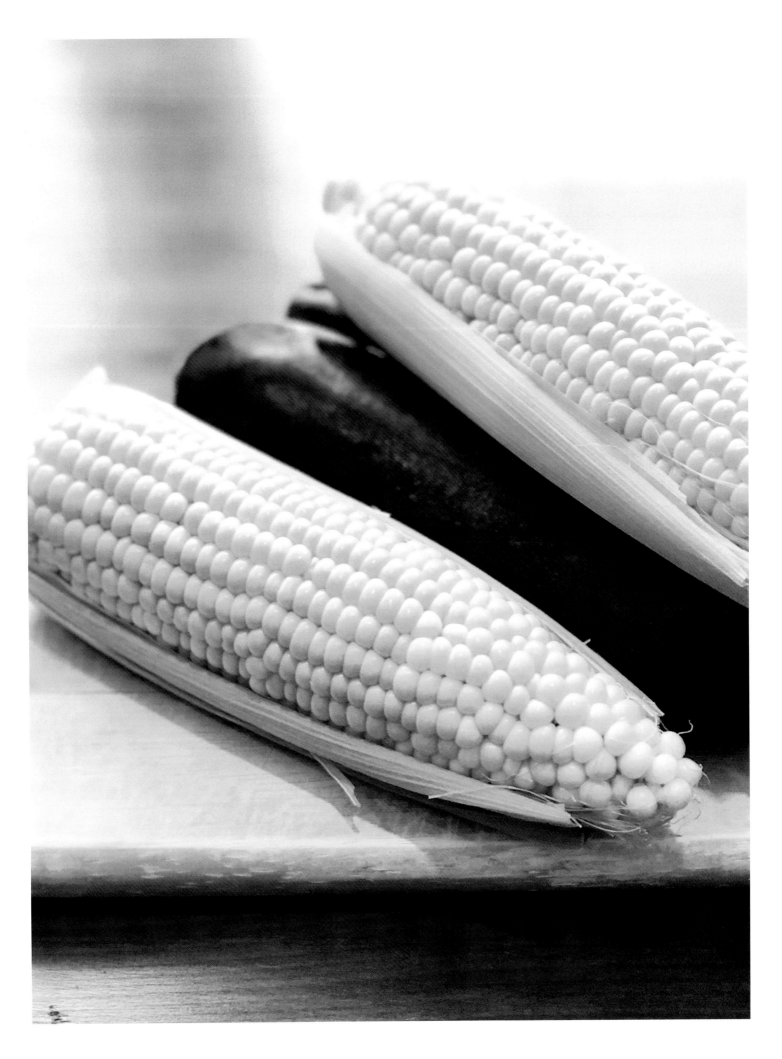

Chili Shrimp & Rice with Mango Jalapeño Sauce

This recipe was a finalist in the Michelle Obama Healthy Lunchtime Cooking Challenge

FOR THE SAUCE:

2 mangoes, peeled, cored, and roughly chopped

½ jalapeño, seeded and roughly minced

6 whole mint leaves

1 tablespoon honey, plus 1 teaspoon after cooked in blender

5 teaspoons water

FOR THE SHRIMP:

¼ teaspoon salt

½ teaspoon pepper

1 teaspoon chili powder

½ teaspoon cumin

4 tablespoons olive oil

30 shrimp, uncooked, peeled and deveined

FOR THE RICE:

3 cups cooked Basmati rice (cooked according to package directions)

1 cup grape tomatoes

Olive oil (as needed)

1 small yellow onion, finely chopped

Salt and pepper (to taste)

½ teaspoon chili powder

1 tablespoon freshly squeezed lemon juice

1 cup fresh pineapple, small diced

1 avocado, medium diced

3-4 medium to small mint leaves, finely chopped and some for garnish

Prepare the sauce: Put the mangoes in a medium sauté pan with the honey and 1 teaspoon water. Cook over medium heat until lightly cooked down, about 10 minutes. Transfer mixture to the blender and blend with jalapeños and mint until smooth. Add 1 teaspoon honey and 4 teaspoons water. Set aside until plating the meal.

Next, cook the rice: Cook rice according to package. Meanwhile, in a separate small sauté pan cook tomatoes with 1 tablespoon olive oil. Season the tomatoes with salt and pepper. Sauté over medium heat until lightly cooked and tender (not popped open). Set aside.

In a medium stockpot over medium heat, sauté the chopped onion with 2 tablespoons olive oil, salt, and pepper to taste. Cook until onions are lightly caramelized (about 10 minutes).

Transfer the cooked rice to the stockpot with the onions in it. Add a splash of olive oil and ½ teaspoon chili powder and mix together. Cook on low heat for 3 minutes.

Add tomatoes to the rice and stir. Turn off heat and cover. Add lemon juice and stir until well mixed.

Right before serving add the chopped pineapple, avocado and mint.

In a small bowl mix all of the spices. Coat the shrimp and set aside. In a large skillet, add 4 tablespoons olive oil and heat pan over medium high heat. Add shrimp and lower heat to medium and cook 4 minutes a side or until fully cooked and pink. Remove from heat.

Plating: On a white plate, pile a big spoonful of rice on one side. Then, line the shrimp up along the inside edge of the rice. Spoon the mango sauce on the remaining space on the plate. Place a bunch of mint leaves in one of the shrimp. Serve warm.

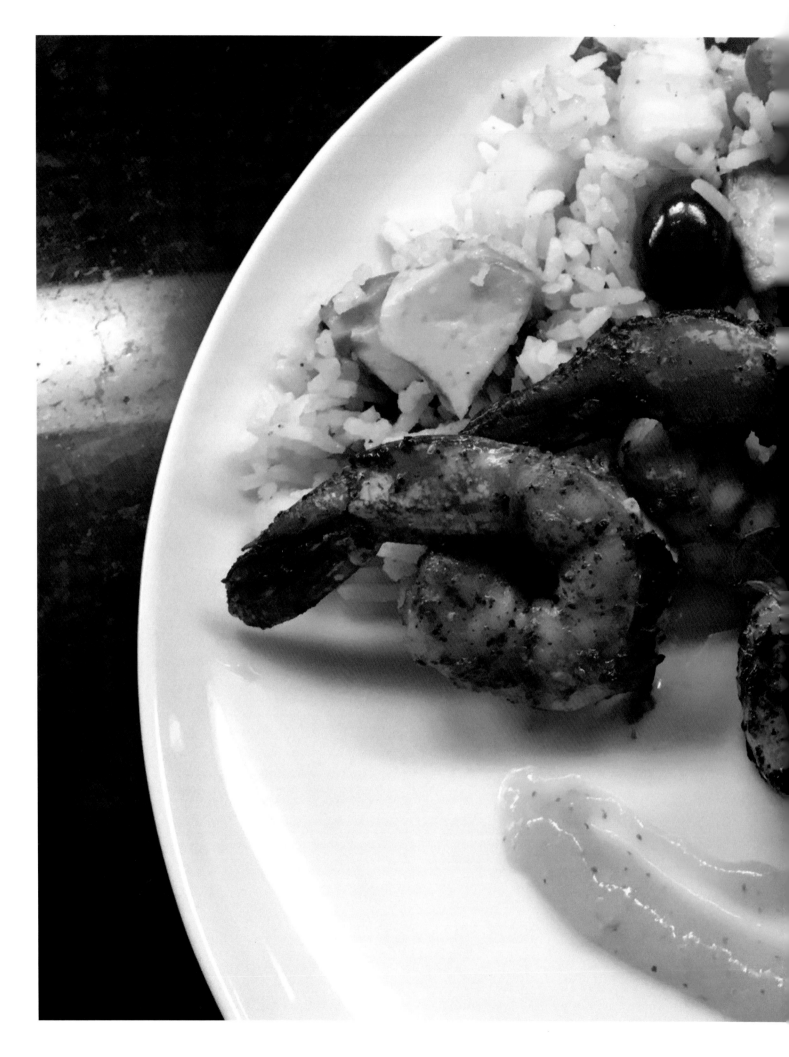

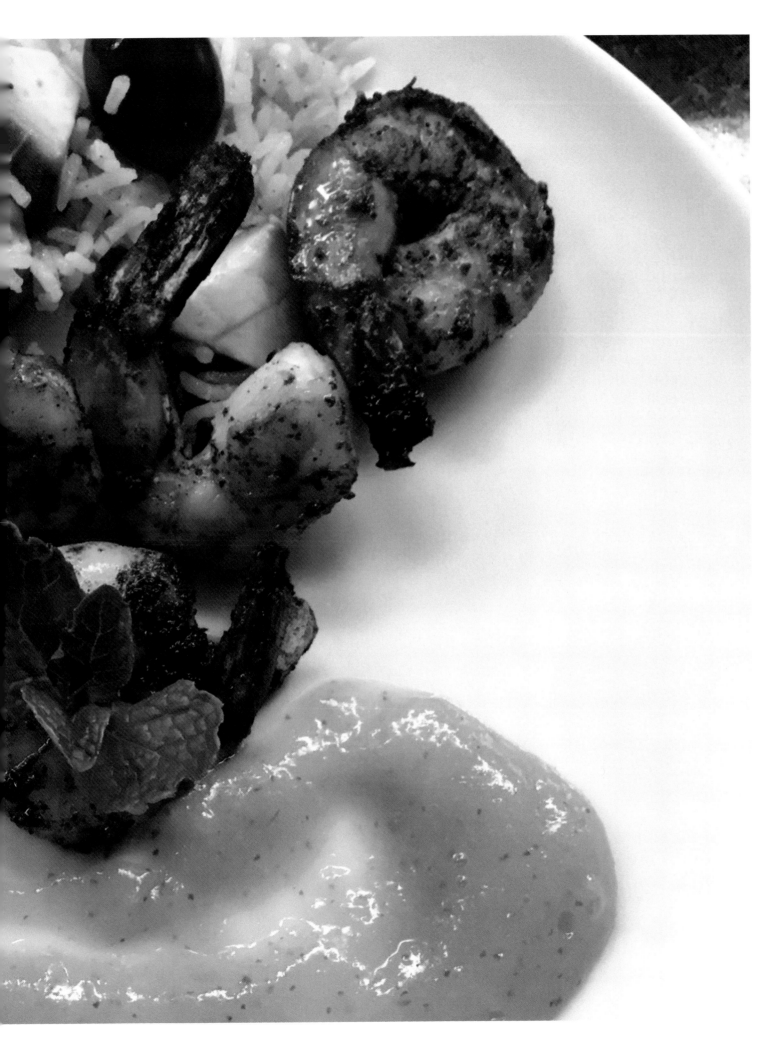

Lemon Baked Cod Fish
with Herb Pesto & Spinach

1½ pounds fresh codfish
Zest of 1 lemon
1 teaspoon lemon juice
Olive oil
Salt and pepper
8 cups fresh spinach, washed

FOR THE PESTO:
1 large handful parsley
3 large basil leaves
1 garlic clove
Olive oil
Zest of 1 lemon
Salt and pepper

Preheat oven to 400°.

On a sheet pan lined with foil place the cod and drizzle with a small amount of olive oil. Add the lemon zest and juice over the cod. Sprinkle with salt and pepper to taste. Bake at 400 degrees for 12 minutes or until white and flaky.

While the fish is cooking assemble the pesto. Place all of the ingredients in a food processor and pulse until finely chopped. Add just the right amount of olive oil to the mixture to make the pesto hold together. Don't over pulse; keep the pesto slightly chunky.

In a large sauté pan, place the spinach and add a small amount of water for steaming the spinach. Cover and cook at medium to low heat until wilted and bright green.

Serve the codfish over the wilted spinach and add pesto on top.

Grilled Halibut with Spinach & Butter Mushrooms

4 fresh halibut steaks (4 ounces each)
4 cups fresh spinach
2 cups chopped baby bello mushrooms
Juice and zest of 1 lemon
2 cloves garlic, minced
2 teaspoons dairy-free butter
1 yellow onion, chopped finely
Salt and pepper

In a large bowl combine the juice and zest with 1 garlic clove and salt and pepper to taste. Place the fish in the bowl with the marinade and let sit for 5 to 10 minutes. Remove the fish from the marinade and grill for 10 minutes or until flaky.

In a sauté pan cook the spinach until wilted but bright green. Add salt and pepper. Set aside.

In another sauté pan cook the mushrooms and onions with the butter and salt and pepper until browned and tender. Add 1 garlic clove and cook for 1 more minute.

Serve halibut with mushroom butter sauce on a bed of the wilted spinach. Squeeze with lemon to taste.

Lemon Sole with Glazed Carrots & Kale Purée

4 fillets Atlantic Sole
Zest of 2 lemons
1 teaspoon freshly squeezed lemon juice
½ teaspoon fresh thyme
32 baby carrots, washed
1 tablespoon dairy-free butter
Olive oil
2 clove garlic, minced
1 tablespoon fresh, chopped chives
2 teaspoons honey
1 large bunch kale
Water (as needed)
Salt
Pepper

Preheat oven to 400°.

On a sheet pan lined with foil, put the fillets of sole on and drizzle with olive oil, lemon juice, sprinkle the zest from 1 lemon, thyme, salt and pepper. Bake in a 400 degree oven for 10 to 12 minutes or until flaky. Serve with the carrots and the sauce.

Boil water in a small pot. Cook the carrots for 3 to 4 minutes, or until they are tender. Transfer the carrots to a sauté pan, add 1 clove of garlic, half of the remaining lemon zest, butter, honey, chives and 1 teaspoon of olive oil. Cook the carrots until soft, or until your liking. Sprinkle with salt and pepper to taste. Serve with the fish.

Blanch the kale in water in a small stock pot. Transfer the kale into a blender (RESERVE KALE WATER). Add the rest of the lemon zest, 1 clove of garlic, salt, pepper, and ½ cup reserved kale water. Blend until smooth. Serve with the fish and carrots.

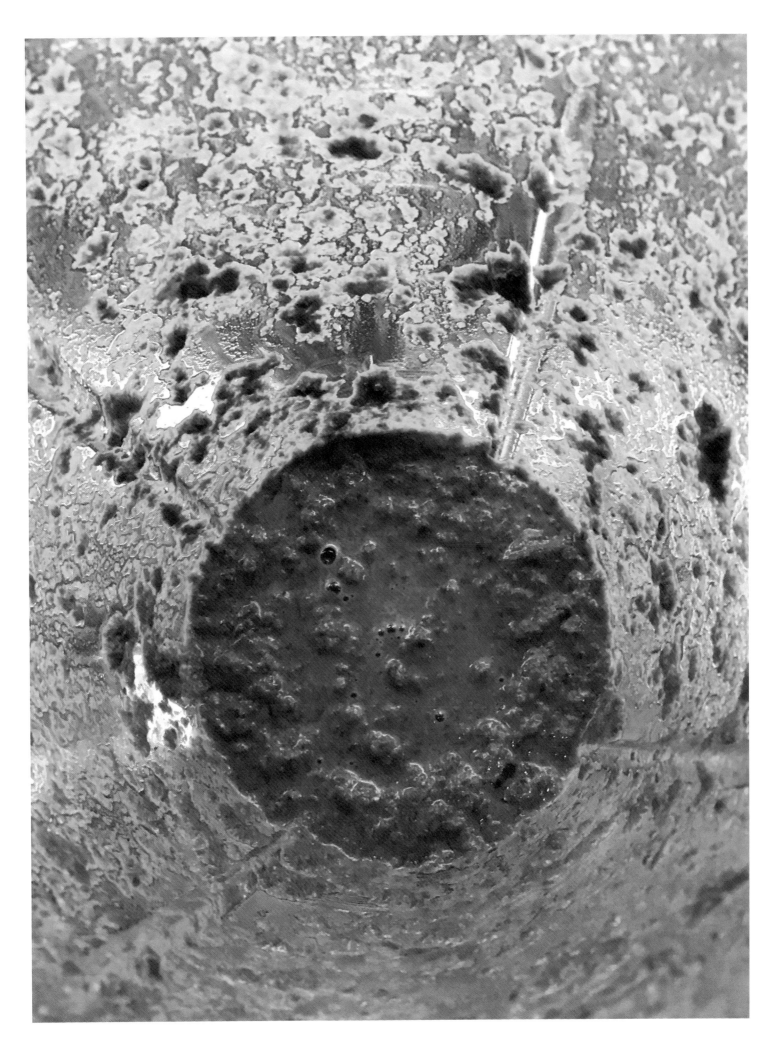

Panko Crusted Cod Fish with Roasted Potatoes & French Green Beans

1½ pounds fresh codfish
1¼ cups Panko breadcrumbs
1 pound red skin potatoes, quartered with skins on
1 pound French green beans
Olive oil
Salt and pepper

Preheat oven to 400°.

On a sheet pan lined with foil, place the potatoes in an even layer and drizzle with olive oil and sprinkle with salt and pepper. Bake at 400 degrees for 35 to 40 minutes or until tender and golden brown.

Combine the Panko with enough olive oil to coat the breadcrumbs. Add salt and pepper to taste.

Place the fish on a sheet pan lined with foil. Sprinkle the breadcrumb mixture over the top of the fish evenly.

Bake at 400 degrees for 12 to 15 minutes or until white and flaky.

While the fish is cooking, blanch the green beans in boiling salted water until bright green and tender.

Cilantro Lime Couscous
with Chipotle Black Beans

FOR THE COUSCOUS:
1 box plain Couscous
2 cups low salt chicken stock
Juice of 1½ limes
2 tablespoons cilantro
1 clove garlic, minced
½ yellow onion, finely chopped
2 tablespoons olive oil

FOR THE DRESSING:
½ cup olive oil
½ teaspoon lime juice
Zest of 1 lime
1 tablespoon fresh cilantro
½ teaspoon chili powder
1 teaspoon red pepper jelly

FOR THE BEANS:
2 cans black beans (14 ounce each), drained
1 tablespoon chipotle pepper, seeded and minced
½ yellow onion, minced
1 teaspoon cumin
1 teaspoon chili powder
¼ teaspoon cayenne pepper
¼ teaspoon coriander
1 teaspoon smoked paprika
1 Roma tomato, small diced
Fresh cilantro
½ cup puréed tomatoes
2 tablespoons olive oil

For the couscous, cook the onions in the 1 tablespoon of olive oil. Boil the chicken stock with the lime juice, lime zest, add the couscous, garlic, and cilantro, turn off heat and cover until the chicken stock is fully absorbed. Stir dressing ingredients together and serve over couscous.

In a small pot heated on medium-high heat, cook the onions in the olive oil until golden brown and caramelized. Add the chopped tomatoes and chipotle pepper and cook for 5 more minutes. Next, add the beans, cumin, chili powder, cayenne, coriander, and paprika. Simmer for 5 to 10 minutes. Then stir in the crushed tomatoes and bring to a boil, cover and then simmer for a while (30 to 45 minutes). Serve warm with the couscous.

Beverages

Non-Alcoholic Blood Orange Cocktail

3 cans 7-Up or Sprite
Juice of 3 blood oranges
3 tablespoons orange juice (fresh or store bought)
Sliced oranges (for garnish)
Ice cubes (as needed)
Mint leaves (for garnish)

Stir everything together in a pitcher. Serve cold with the garnishes and ice.

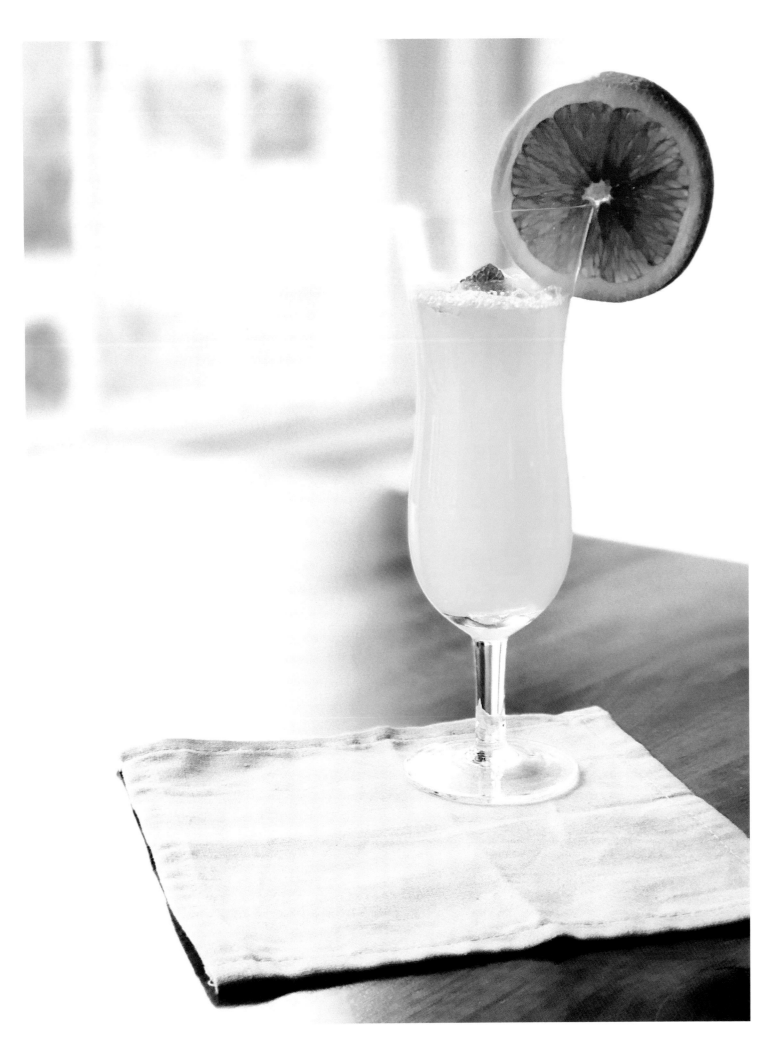

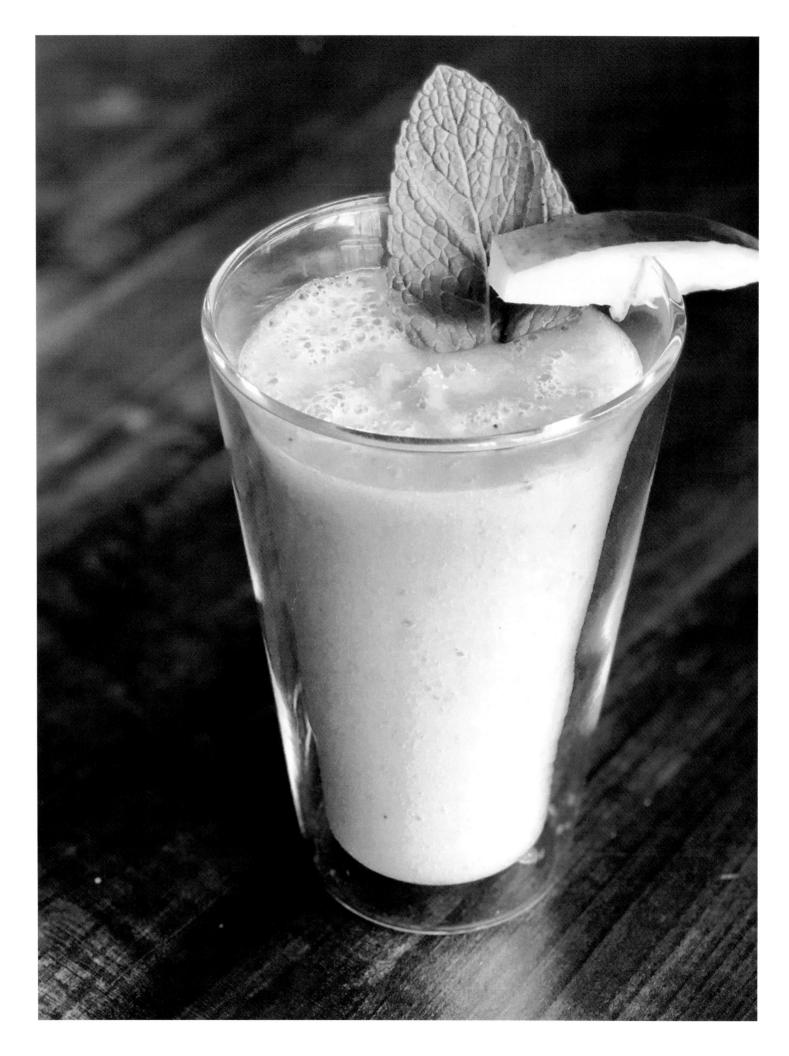

Tropical Paradise Smoothie

½ cup frozen or fresh mangoes
2 bananas
1 ounce pineapple juice
1 peach, cut into slices
Zest of 1 orange
1-1½ cups dairy-free milk
1 tablespoon orange juice

Blend everything in a blender. Serve cold.

Peppermint Hot Chocolate

4 cups soy or rice milk
4 tablespoons chocolate syrup
½ teaspoon peppermint extract

In a large saucepan combine all of the ingredients over low heat until desired temperature. Serve warm with marshmallows and a peppermint stick.

Lemon Herb Iced Tea

6 cups water
6 Lipton tea bags
10 mint leaves
Juice of 1 lemon
Thin lemon slices, seeded
¼ cup sugar
Ice

In a large stock pot, add the water and bring to a boil. Then add the sugar and dissolve it before continuing. Next, add the tea bags and half of the mint and lemon juice. Cover and steep for 10 minutes. Strain the mixture and discard the tea bags and leaves.

Chill and serve over ice garnished with mint and lemon slices.

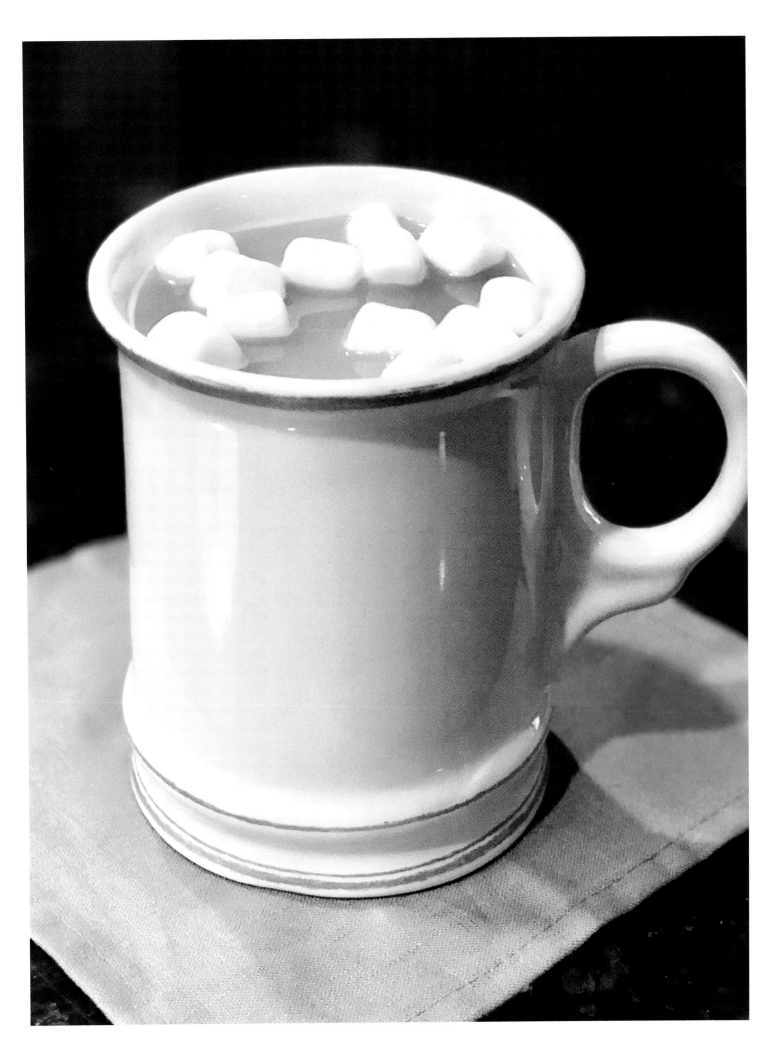

Desserts

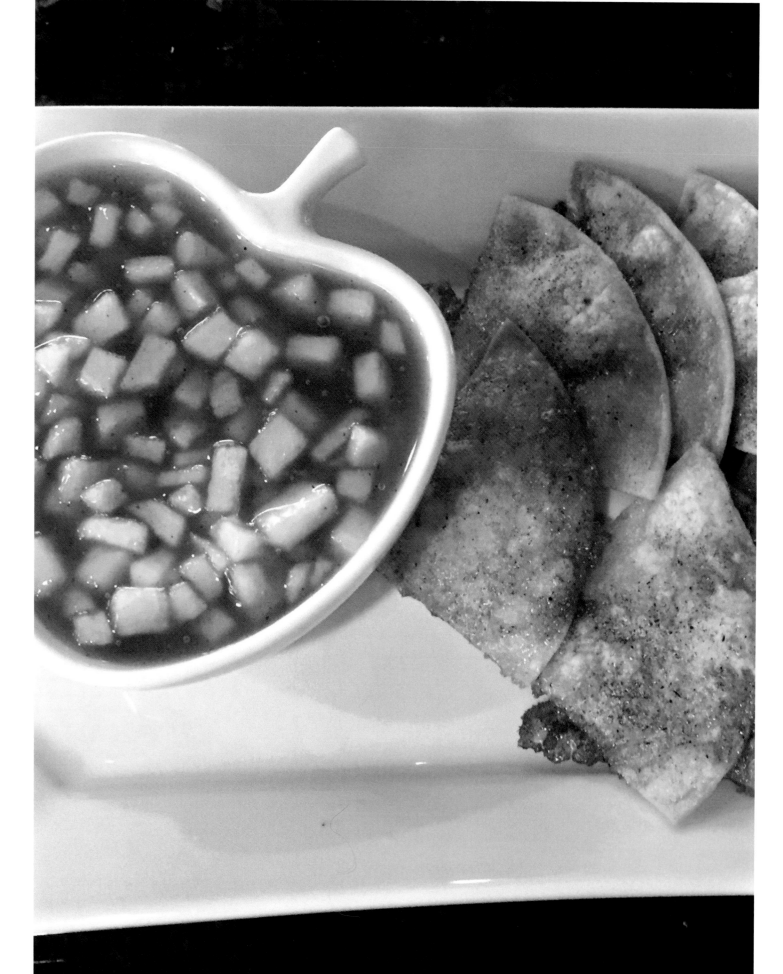

Cinnamon Crisps with Warm Apple Compote

FOR THE CRISPS:
8 corn tortillas (cut into fourths)
5 tablespoons granulated sugar
1 teaspoon cinnamon
6 tablespoons canola oil

FOR THE COMPOTE:
3 apples (ones that are good for baking)
⅓ cup warm water
2 teaspoons cornstarch
1 teaspoon cinnamon
½ cup plus 1 teaspoon granulated sugar

Preheat oven to 350°.

Make the crisps: Lay out the tortillas on a sheet pan covered in foil, in one layer. Drizzle with the oil. Then, generously sprinkle with the sugar and cinnamon. Bake at 350 degrees until golden brown and crisp (11 to 13 minutes). Serve warm with apple compote.

Make the compote: Cube the apples and transfer into a small pot. Turn the stove on at medium heat. Add the water, cornstarch, and sugar, stir until thick. Add the cinnamon and let simmer on low until apples are cooked through (stirring often). Transfer into serving dish and serve warm with the crisps.

Fragrant Lemon Cake

FOR THE CAKE:
1 cup plus 1 tablespoon sugar
1 cup flour
½ teaspoon baking soda
½ cup canola oil
1 cup plus 1 tablespoon rice milk
1¼ tablespoons vinegar
Zest of 1½– 2 lemons
¼ teaspoon salt

FOR THE GLAZE:
2 cups confectioner sugar
4 tablespoons rice milk
¼ teaspoon vanilla extract
Zest of 1-½ lemons

Preheat oven to 375º.

Sift together the flour, baking soda, and salt. In a mixer, mix the milk, vinegar, lemon zest, canola oil, and sugar. Slowly add the flour mixture to the wet ingredients. Mix until there are no lumps. Transfer to a 9 by 9 circular cake pan. Bake for 20 to 22 minutes or until a toothpick comes out clean. Cool. Serve with the lemon glaze following.

In a mixer, combine the sugar, milk, vanilla, and lemon. Mix until it is smooth. Serve over the lemon cake. Chill the leftovers in the fridge.

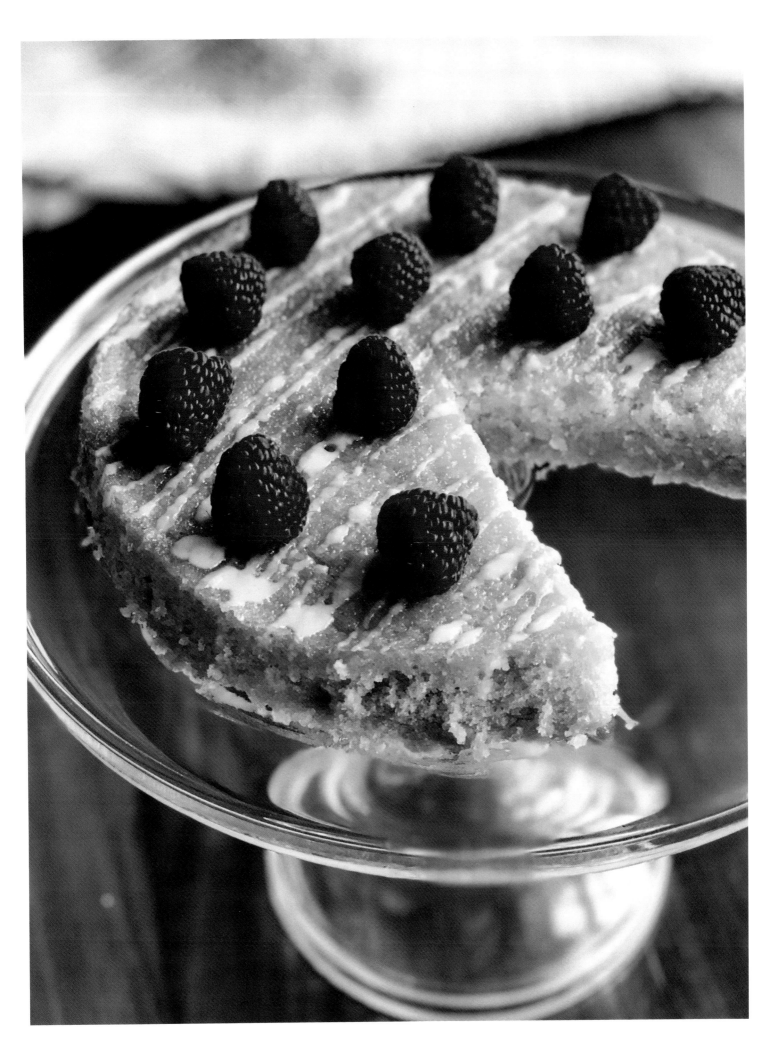

Maple Brown Sugar Pastries

FOR THE SAUCE:
⅔ cup pure maple syrup
¼ cup brown sugar
1 teaspoon granulated sugar
1 tablespoon water

FOR THE PASTRY:
1 package puff pastry
½ cup brown sugar
1 tablespoon dairy-free butter

Preheat oven to 350°.

Make the sauce: Heat all of the ingredients in a saucepan on medium heat. Cook until smooth. Drizzle over the pastries.

Prepare the pastry: Melt the butter in the microwave and set aside for later. Roll out the puff pastry and with a pastry cutter, cut into squares. Set aside half of the squares. Sprinkle the other half with brown sugar. Take the squares that were set aside, and put them on top of the squares with brown sugar. Seal the pastries by pressing them with a fork all the way around. Brush each pastry with the melted butter, and sprinkle with sugar. Cook about 10 to 15 minutes or until golden brown. Serve warm with the sauce.

Blueberry Pastries

FOR THE PASTRY:
1 package puff pastry
Powdered sugar

FOR THE SAUCE:
Juice of 1 lemon
2 tablespoons granulated sugar
2½ cups frozen blueberries
¼ cup water

Preheat oven to 350°.

Roll the puff pastry out on a board. Cut the puff pastry with a 1 inch by 1 inch circular or square cookie cutter. Put them on a sheet pan lined with foil. You will have approximately 75 pastries.

Bake them at 350 degrees for 15 to 20 minutes or until golden brown and crisp. Dust with powdered sugar. Serve warm.

Put the berries in a simmering pot with the water, sugar, and lemon juice. Let everything cook down until lightly bubbling. Serve warm with the pastries.

Warm Blueberry Crisp

1½ pints fresh blueberries, washed and drained
Zest of 1 lemon
Juice of 1 lemon
1 tablespoon freshly squeezed orange juice
3 tablespoons granulated sugar
3 tablespoons all-purpose flour
⅛ teaspoon cinnamon

FOR THE TOPPING:
1 cup rolled oats
¾ cup brown sugar
2 tablespoons all-purpose flour
1 tablespoon granulated sugar
3 tablespoons dairy-free butter
1 teaspoon honey

Preheat oven to 350°.

In a medium bowl toss the blueberries, lemon zest, lemon juice, orange juice, sugar, flour, and cinnamon until the blueberries are fully coated in the mixture. Set aside.

Combine all of topping ingredients in a medium bowl. Then in a pie dish press half of the topping on the bottom of the dish. Add the blueberry mixture and then sprinkle with the remaining topping. Bake at 350 degrees for 30 to 35 minutes until bubbly and golden brown on top. Remove from oven and cool for around 10 minutes. Serve warm with dairy-free vanilla ice cream.

Blueberry Syrup

2 bags frozen blueberries
1 cup granulated sugar
2 teaspoons cornstarch
¼ cup water

Place the blueberries in a small pot with ¼ cup water. Simmer. Add the sugar and cornstarch and stir. Cook on medium heat until bubbling. Turn off heat and strain in a strainer to separate the whole blueberries. (The whole blueberries can be used if you want).

Let the sauce cool for 10 to 15 minutes until thick. Serve on top of pancakes, waffles, ice cream, yogurt, or anything that you want. Chill.

Vanilla Ice Cream Pie

1 tub dairy-free vanilla ice cream
1 Oreo chocolate pie crust

Thaw the ice cream and transfer to the pie crust.
Chill until the ice cream is set. Serve cold.

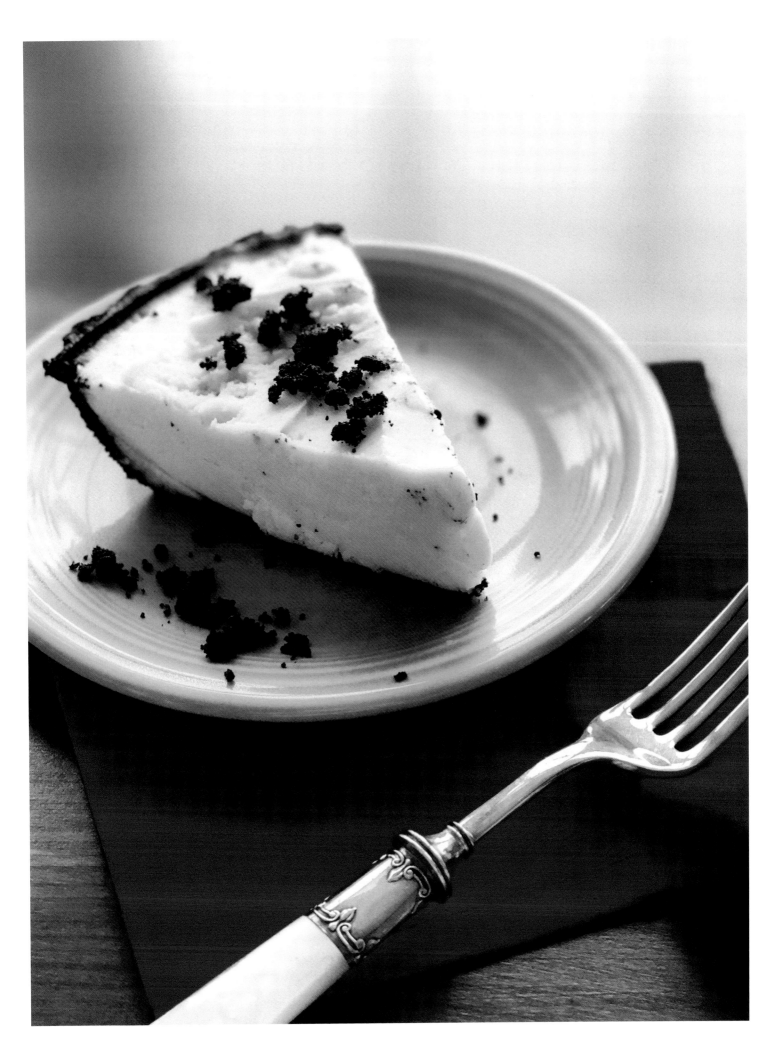

Cinnamon Sugar Swirl Ice Cream

1 tub dairy-free vanilla ice cream
½ cup light brown sugar
1 teaspoon cinnamon
1 tablespoon dark brown sugar

Let the ice cream soften first. In a large bowl stir in the brown sugars and the cinnamon to the ice cream. Freeze back in the tub. Let it thaw at least 5 to 10 minutes before serving.

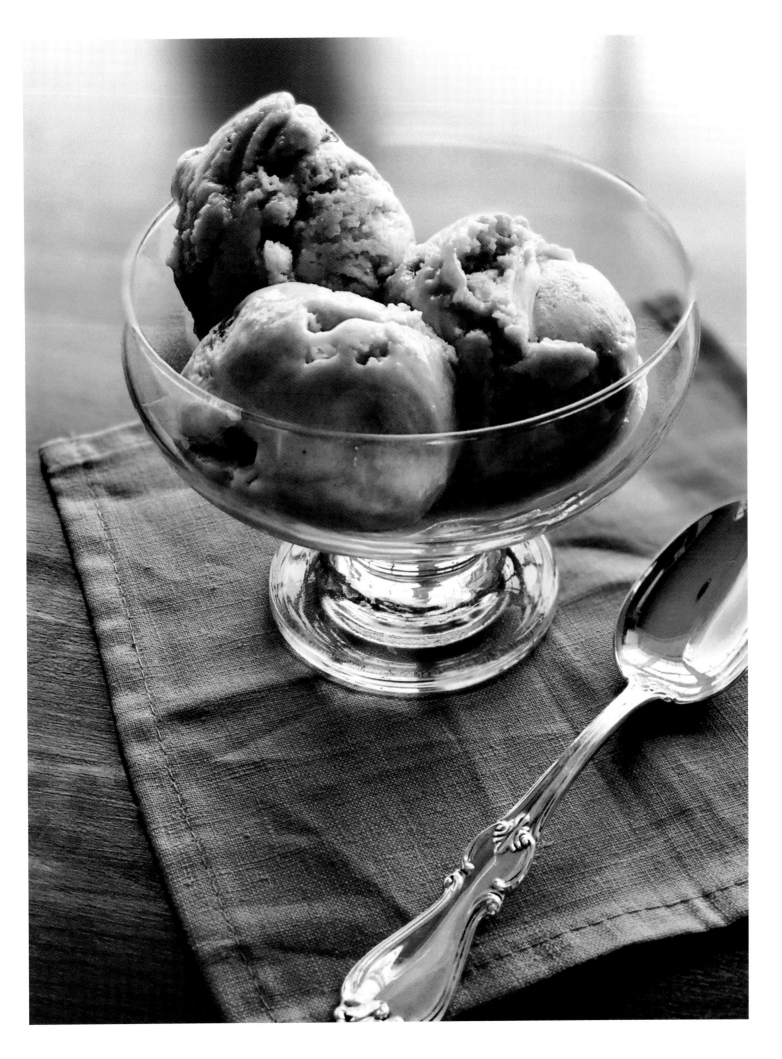

Mint Chocolate Chip Ice Cream

1 tub dairy-free vanilla ice cream
½-1 teaspoon peppermint extract
1½ cups mini dairy-free chocolate chips

Let the ice cream thaw out until it is soft. Transfer it into a large bowl, stir in the peppermint and chocolate chips. Transfer back into the tub of ice cream or a Tupperware container. Freeze. Let it sit out for at least 5 to 10 minutes before serving.

French Toast Made Easy

(V)

¾ cup dairy-free milk
1 tablespoon brown sugar
½ teaspoon vanilla
⅛ teaspoon cinnamon
4 slices white bread
1 tablespoon dairy-free butter

Whisk together the milk, sugar, vanilla, and cinnamon. Meanwhile heat a small skillet on medium with 1 teaspoon of the butter. Brush the bread with the wet mixture. Set in heated pan. Cook until golden brown and crisp. Serve with berries or maple syrup.

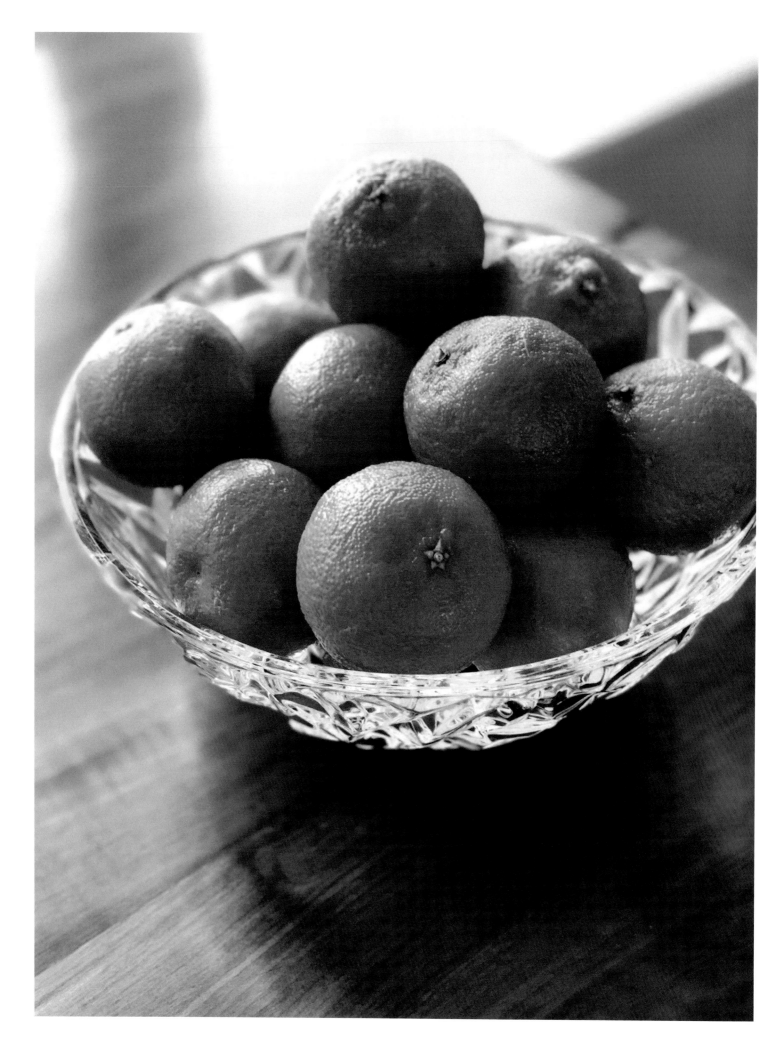

Index